Mental Health Issues of Older Women: A Comprehensive Review for Health Care Professionals

Mental Health Issues of Older Women: A Comprehensive Review for Health Care Professionals has been co-published simultaneously as *Journal of Women & Aging*, Volume 19, Numbers 1/2 2007.

Monographic Separates from the *Journal of Women & Aging*®

For additional information on these and other Haworth Press titles, including descriptions, tables of contents, reviews, and prices, use the QuickSearch catalog at http://www.HaworthPress.com.

Mental Health Issues of Older Women: A Comprehensive Review for Health Care Professionals, edited by Victor J. Malatesta, PhD (Vol. 19, No. 1/2, 2007). *Comprehensive overview of the latest research and current issues on the mental health problems of older women.*

Widows and Divorcees in Later Life: On Their Own Again, edited by Carol L. Jenkins, MPA, PhD (Vol. 15, No. 2/3, 2003). *"Exhaustive. . . . Richly textured. . . . This book may well emerge as a seminal work on this topic." (David K. Brown, PhD, Associate Director, Center on Aging, West Virginia University)*

Health Expectations for Older Women: International Perspectives, edited by Sarah B. Laditka, PhD (Vol. 14, No. 1/2, 2002). *"Brings together noted experts from around the world who shed new light on how women age. . . . This volume is sweeping in its coverage, including specific analyses of the U.S., the U.K., Japan, Canada, The Netherlands, and Fiji, as well as an overview of all 191 WHO member countries. A nice balance of country-specific and global studies. . . . Gerontologists, epidemiologists, and demographers will find the information presented to be timely, rigorous, and accessible." (Christine L. Himes, PhD, Associate Professor of Sociology, Syracuse University)*

Fundamentals of Feminist Gerontology, edited by J. Dianne Garner, DSW (Vol. 11, No. 2/3, 1999). *Strives to increase women's self-esteem and their overall quality of life by encouraging education and putting a stop to age, sex, and race discrimination.*

Old, Female, and Rural, edited by B. Jan McCulloch (Vol. 10, No. 4, 1998). *"An excellent job of bringing together experts from four different disciplines to illuminate the basic interdisciplinary nature of gerontology." (Dr. Jean Turner, Associate Professor, Human Development and Family Services, University of Arkansas, Fayetteville, Arkansas)*

Relationships Between Women in Later Life, edited by Karen A. Roberto (Vol. 8, No. 3/4, 1996). *"Provides an impressive array of issues about women's social networks. . . . Important, up-to-date empirical studies that will fill a significant gap in our understanding about the great diversity in the lives of older women today." (European Federation of the Elderly)*

Older Women with Chronic Pain, edited by Karen A. Roberto (Vol. 6, No. 4, 1994). *"Readers interested in the health concerns of older women, and older women themselves, will appreciate the insight and information in this book." (Feminist Bookstore News)*

Women and Healthy Aging: Living Productively in Spite of It All, edited by J. Dianne Garner and Alice A. Young (Vol. 5, No. 3/4, 1994). *"For those who are not aged themselves, it helps to bring about insights that are not possible when one holds the commonly taught view that disability of any degree is strictly debilitating." (Linda Vinton, PhD, Associate Professor, School of Social Work, Florida State University; Research Affiliate, Pepper Institute on Aging and Public Policy)*

Women in Mid-Life: Planning for Tomorrow, edited by Christopher L. Hayes (Vol. 4, No. 4, 1993). *"Contains illuminating insights into aspects of women's mid-life experiences." (Age and Ageing)*

Women, Aging and Ageism, edited by Evelyn Rosenthal (Vol. 2, No. 2, 1990). *"Readers should find this book helpful in gaining new insights to issues women face in old age . . . Enlightening." (Educational Gerontology)*

Women as They Age: Challenge, Opportunity, and Triumph, edited by J. Dianne Garner and Susan O. Mercer (Vol. 1, No. 1/2/3, 1989). *"Offers provocative insights into the strengths, dilemmas, and challenges confronting the current and future cohorts of older women." (Affilia: Journal of Women and Social Work)*

Mental Health Issues of Older Women: A Comprehensive Review for Health Care Professionals

Victor J. Malatesta, PhD

Editor

Mental Health Issues of Older Women: A Comprehensive Review for Health Care Professionals has been co-published simultaneously as *Journal of Women & Aging*, Volume 19, Numbers 1/2 2007.

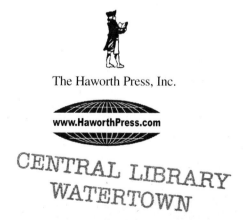

The Haworth Press, Inc.

www.HaworthPress.com

Mental Health Issues of Older Women: A Comprehensive Review for Health Care Professionals has been co-published simultaneously as *Journal of Women & Aging*®, Volume 19, Numbers 1/2 2007.

The development, preparation, and publication of this work has been undertaken with great care. However, the publisher, employees, editors, and agents of The Haworth Press and all imprints of The Haworth Press, Inc., including The Haworth Medical Press® and Pharmaceutical Products Press®, are not responsible for any errors contained herein or for consequences that may ensue from use of materials or information contained in this work. With regard to case studies, identities and circumstances of individuals discussed herein have been changed to protect confidentiality. Any resemblance to actual persons, living or dead, is entirely coincidental.

The Haworth Press is committed to the dissemination of ideas and information according to the highest standards of intellectual freedom and the free exchange of ideas. Statements made and opinions expressed in this publication do not necessarily reflect the views of the Publisher, Directors, management, or staff of The Haworth Press, Inc., or an endorsement by them.

Cover design by Kerry E. Mack

Library of Congress Cataloging-in-Publication Data

Mental health issues of older women : a comprehensive review for health care professionals / Victor J. Malatesta, editor.
    p. cm.
    "Co-published simultaneously as Journal of women & aging, volume 19, numbers 1/2, 2007."
    Includes bibliographical references and index.
    ISBN-13: 978-0-7890-3597-4 (hard cover : alk. paper)
    ISBN-10: 0-7890-3597-9 (hard cover : alk. paper)
    ISBN-13: 978-0-7890-3598-1 (soft cover : alk. paper)
    ISBN-10: 0-7890-3598-7 (soft cover : alk. paper)
    1. Older women–Mental health. 2. Middle-aged women–Mental health. I. Malatesta, Victor J. (Victor Julio)
  [DNLM: 1. Mental Disorders. 2. Aged. 3. Middle Aged. 4. Women–psychology. W1 JO972H v.19 no.1/2 2007 / WT 150 M54945 2007]
  RC451.4.A5M457 2007
  362.2082–dc22

                                                  2006031523

The HAWORTH PRESS *Inc.*
Abstracting, Indexing & Outward Linking
PRINT *and* ELECTRONIC BOOKS & JOURNALS

This section provides you with a list of major indexing & abstracting services and other tools for bibliographic access. That is to say, each service began covering this periodical during the the year noted in the right column. Most Websites which are listed below have indicated that they will either post, disseminate, compile, archive, cite or alert their own Website users with research-based content from this work. (This list is as current as the copyright date of this publication.)

Abstracting, Website/Indexing Coverage . . . . Year When Coverage Began

- **Academic ASAP (Thomson Gale)** 1992
- **Academic Search Premier (EBSCO)* *
  <http://search.ebscohost.com>. 1996
- **CINAHL (Cumulative Index to Nursing & Allied Health
  Literature) (EBSCO)** <http://www.cinahl.com> 1996
- **CINAHL Plus (EBSCO)** <http://search.ebscohost.com> 2006
- **Current Contents/Social & Behavioral Sciences (Thomson
  Scientific)** <http://www.isinet.com> 1995
- **Expanded Academic ASAP (Thomson Gale)** 1992
- **Expanded Academic ASAP–International (Thomson Gale)**. . . . 1992
- **InfoTrac Custom (Thomson Gale)** 1992
- **InfoTrac OneFile (Thomson Gale)** 1992
- **Journal Citation Reports/Social Sciences Edition (Thomson
  Scientific)** <http://www.isinet.com> 2005
- **MEDLINE (National Library of Medicine)**
  <http://www.nlm.nih.gov> 1999
- **ProQuest Academic Research Library**
  <http://www.proquest.com>. 2006
- **Psychological Abstracts (PsycINFO)* * <http://www.apa.org> . . . 2001
- **PubMed** <http://www.ncbi.nlm.nih.gov/pubmed> 1999
- **Research Library (ProQuest)** <http://www.proquest.com>. 2006

(continued)

(continued)

(continued)

(continued)

Bibliographic Access

Special Bibliographic Notes related to special journal issues (separates) and indexing/abstracting:

- indexing/abstracting services in this list will also cover material in any "separate" that is co-published simultaneously with Haworth's special thematic journal issue or DocuSerial. Indexing/abstracting usually covers material at the article/chapter level.
- monographic co-editions are intended for either non-subscribers or libraries which intend to purchase a second copy for their circulating collections.
- monographic co-editions are reported to all jobbers/wholesalers/approval plans. The source journal is listed as the "series" to assist the prevention of duplicate purchasing in the same manner utilized for books-in-series.
- to facilitate user/access services all indexing/abstracting services are encouraged to utilize the co-indexing entry note indicated at the bottom of the first page of each article/chapter/contribution.
- this is intended to assist a library user of any reference tool (whether print, electronic, online, or CD-ROM) to locate the monographic version if the library has purchased this version but not a subscription to the source journal.
- individual articles/chapters in any Haworth publication are also available through The Haworth Document Delivery Service (HDDS).

As part of Haworth's continuing committment to better serve our library patrons, we are proud to be working with the following electronic services:

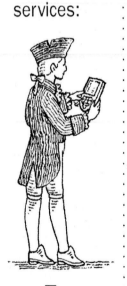

AGGREGATOR SERVICES

EBSCOhost

Ingenta

J-Gate

Minerva

OCLC FirstSearch

Oxmill

SwetsWise

FirstSearch

Oxmill Publishing
SwetsWise

LINK RESOLVER SERVICES

1Cate (Openly Informatics)

CrossRef

Gold Rush (Coalliance)

LinkOut (PubMed)

LINKplus (Atypon)

LinkSolver (Ovid)

LinkSource with A-to-Z (EBSCO)

Resource Linker (Ulrich)

SerialsSolutions (ProQuest)

SFX (Ex Libris)

Sirsi Resolver (SirsiDynix)

Tour (TDnet)

Vlink (Extensity, *formerly Geac*)

WebBridge (Innovative Interfaces)

Gold Rush

LinkOut.
LINKING TO A WORLD OF RESOURCES

atypon
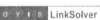
LinkSolver

ULRICH'S RESOURCE LINKER
$S \cdot F \cdot X$
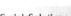
SerialsSolutions

SirsiDynix
TOUR

((extensity))

WebBridge

Mental Health Issues of Older Women: A Comprehensive Review for Health Care Professionals

CONTENTS

ABOUT THE EDITOR

Victor J. Malatesta, PhD, is a licensed psychologist who maintains a practice in clinical psychology and neuropsychology in West Chester and Wynnewood, PA. He is a clinical Associate Professor of Psychology in the Department of Psychiatry, University of Pennsylvania School of Medicine, and an adjunct member of the professional staff of Pennsylvania Hospital. He received his training at the University of Delaware, University of Georgia, and the Consortium of the Medical University of South Carolina/Charleston Veterans Administration Medical Center. In 1980, Dr. Malatesta received one of the first certificates in gerontology (of which he is most proud) from the University of Georgia's Program on Gerontology. His published work in the field of gerontology has included the neuropsychology of aging, adaptation to widowhood, and human sexuality across the life span. He has published over 50 scientific articles and book chapters and he has been a consultant to agencies on aging, including the National Council on Aging. His clinical interests include behavioral psychotherapy with adults and older adults and couples. Dr. Malatesta was honored by Philadelphia Magazine as one of the Top Doctors for Women.

Acknowledgments

This project is dedicated to the women in my life who have loved, challenged, encouraged and inspired me, both personally and professionally. To my wife, Caryn Malatesta, MA, RN, who offered special support and handled some of the writing and editing; to my daughter Jessa who provided much needed computer consultation and data management services; to my mother, Gloria Faenza Malatesta, for inspiration and instilling in me an interest and respect for all individuals; to my mother-in-law, Marcine Davis, for love and support; to Dianne Chambless, PhD, who was my first woman supervisor and who offered her clinical wisdom and raised my consciousness about the importance of women's issues; to Patricia B. Sutker, PhD, who was my internship supervisor and who shared her keen research mind and scholarly writing habits; to Judy Saltzberg, PhD, colleague and friend, for sharing such a great work environment; and a special thanks to Dianne Garner, DSW, Editor of the *Journal of Women & Aging,* for offering me this opportunity and for providing expert guidance and encouragement throughout the project. I also want to thank each of the authors for their excellent contributions–without which this project would not have been possible. Finally, this project is dedicated to our older women clients and patients who have allowed us to witness their courage, tenacity and grace as they negotiate this incredible process called aging.

Introduction:
The Need to Address Older Women's
Mental Health Issues

Victor J. Malatesta, PhD

SUMMARY. Women are the primary consumers of mental health services. Ironically, research addressing their unique needs lags behind that of men's issues. The aging process introduces an important variable that accentuates the relative lack of information and specific treatment guidelines for older women who are confronted by mental health problems. This volume offers a comprehensive overview for the health professional who is seeking a greater depth of understanding with respect to the study of mental health problems in general, and how these issues pertain specifically to women and the aging process. A second goal of this project is to provide the practicing therapist and counselor with a research update and a broad clinical perspective offered by seasoned clinicians. Using current psychiatric diagnosis as a framework, the contributions address the range of mental health problems, including dementia and cognitive impairment, schizophrenia, alcohol abuse, mood and anxiety disorders, traumatic and dissociative conditions, sexual and eating disorders, and personality disorders. It is hoped that this book will inform, inspire and encourage students and health professionals in their work with middle aged and older women who are facing mental health challenges. doi:10.1300/J074v19n01_01 *[Article copies available for a fee from The Haworth Document Delivery Service: 1-800-HAWORTH. E-mail address: <docdelivery@haworthpress.com> Website: <http://www.HaworthPress. com> © 2007 by The Haworth Press, Inc. All rights reserved.]*

[Haworth co-indexing entry note]: "Introduction: The Need to Address Older Women's Mental Health Issues." Malatesta, Victor J. Co-published simultaneously in *Journal of Women & Aging* (The Haworth Press, Inc.) Vol. 19, No. 1/2, 2007, pp. 1-12; and: *Mental Health Issues of Older Women: A Comprehensive Review for Health Care Professionals* (ed: Victor J. Malatesta) The Haworth Press, Inc., 2007, pp. 1-12. Single or multiple copies of this article are available for a fee from The Haworth Document Delivery Service [1-800-HAWORTH, 9:00 a.m. - 5:00 p.m. (EST). E-mail address: docdelivery@haworthpress.com].

KEYWORDS. Women, mental health, aging, psychopathology, mental illness

Women are the primary consumers of mental health services. Ironically, research addressing their unique needs lags far behind that of men's issues. It is only recently that medicine has recognized that women have different health needs and require specially tailored evaluation and treatment services. As a consequence, women are receiving more research and clinical attention, and there is a new focus on traditionally male dominated health issues, such as cardiac care and cancer treatment (Hobson, 2006). With respect to mental health needs, however, the gender imbalance is more striking. For example, while women are much more likely to suffer from depression, use psychotropic medication and seek the services of a mental health professional, the bulk of available clinical and research studies, until recently, has tended to focus on men as subjects. In addition, there are certain clinical and research areas that reflect a long-standing disparity in favor of men (e.g., treatment of sexual problems). Although the situation has improved dramatically (e.g., Hughes, Smith, & Dan, 2003; Slater, Daniel, & Banks, 2003; Trotman & Brody, 2002), there continues to be a relative dearth in our research and clinical knowledge of women's mental health issues.

MENTAL HEALTH AND THE AGING PROCESS

The aging process represents an important variable that exerts a diverse and profound effect on the mental health status of women and men alike. For example, estimates suggest that approximately 20% of older adults have a mental disorder (Gatz & Smyer, 2001). Yet, mental health services are underutilized by older adults who are more likely to present their mental health needs to their primary care physicians within the context of physical illness (Mickus & Colenda, 2000). Similarly, the U.S. Surgeon General has recognized that disability due to late-life mental illness is a major public health concern for the 21st century (U.S. Surgeon General, DHHS, 1999). Although there is a great need for mental health research on aging in general (see Knight et al., 1995), there is relatively less that we know about older women, and how they negotiate the aging process with respect to their mental health needs.

There are several reasons why the study of older women's mental health is an important and worthy endeavor. In this volume, you will learn that:

1. Middle aged and older women live significantly longer than their male counterparts and, as a consequence, are more likely to develop a chronic illness, including dementia;
2. Because of their greater longevity, older women are more likely to experience a range of losses, including those associated with their health, their family, and their support system;
3. Because of multiple factors, older women are more likely to suffer a range of psychosocial stressors associated with their living status, unemployment and inadequate income, relocation, and access to services;
4. Older women are subject to a wide diversity of racial, ethnic, and sociocultural influences that are inadequately understood by health professionals and which complicate identification of their needs and delivery of services (see Hinrichsen, 2006);
5. Older women are more likely than older men to develop an anxiety disorder, suffer from depression, and experience post traumatic reactions, including dissociative disorder;
6. Certain mental health problems, such as alcohol abuse and prescription medication abuse, are especially underdiagnosed in older women; yet,
7. Middle aged and older women are more likely to function as long-term caregivers for their children, their partners, and their parents–sometimes while also remaining employed;
8. Older women have a greater likelihood of utilizing assisted living services and long-term nursing care; and,
9. In conjunction with these above findings, it has also been reported that many older adults, including women, report greater levels of contentment than at any time in their lives, suggesting that exposure to a lifetime of inevitable challenges and stressors may result in a special resiliency and enhanced coping abilities (see Fisher et al., 2001).

With these points in mind, the purpose of this special collection is to provide a comprehensive overview for the health professional who is seeking a greater depth of understanding with respect to the study of mental health issues in general, and how they pertain specifically to women and the aging process. A second goal of this project is to provide the practicing therapist and counselor with a research update and a comprehensive clinical perspective offered by seasoned clinicians. Each article attempts to provide a scholarly blend of scientific and practical information. For each mental health disorder, the authors–the majority of whom work primarily in clinical settings–sought to include current information about description and diagnosis, based upon the current and most widely utilized psychiatric classification scheme (DSM-IV-TR: Diagnostic and Statistical Manual of Mental Disorders, 4th Edition, Text Revision, American Psychiatric Association, 2000). In addition, issues of prevalence, etiology, assessment and treatment were included. The authors also attempted to address special issues associated with the female aging process in particular, including menopause, the role of medical illness, loss and bereavement, and psychosocial characteristics. Finally, the authors emphasize areas of need for future research and additional study.

THE STUDY OF PSYCHOPATHOLOGY
IN LATER ADULTHOOD

The study of mental health problems is known formally as the study of psychopathology (Adams, 1981). The field of psychopathology is based first upon a thorough and comprehensive understanding of normal behavior and its patterns. From this vantage point, the study of psychopathology aims to describe, classify and understand abnormal behavior from a broad etiological perspective where possible (see Adams & Sutker, 2001). Attending to biological, psychological and sociocultural factors, a multifaceted biopsychosocial approach is often implied. Ultimately, the study of psychopathology provides a foundation from which to address issues of diagnosis, assessment, treatment, and future research.

In addressing the relationship between psychopathology, aging and women, we attempted to examine it from three perspectives, including (1) mental health problems that may develop for the first time in middle and later adulthood; (2) disorders that are first displayed in adolescence or early adulthood and continue during the later years, and either remain unchanged or are altered by the aging process; and (3) mental disorders that begin in early or middle adulthood and tend to attenuate or remit. To a varying degree, each of these three perspectives is reflected in each article, depending upon the nature of the topic. One important finding is that the reader will observe that, while there are many similarities between older men and women, there are also marked gender differences in mental health problems among older adults. Similarly, the reader will appreciate that the female life course of psychopathology, in contrast to the male perspective, may be quite different depending upon the disorder under study. The differences have implications for needs identification, assessment, design of effective treatment interventions, and overall service delivery.

THREE KEY CONCEPTS IN STUDYING THE MENTAL HEALTH ISSUES OF OLDER WOMEN

Variability (Diversity) Increases with Age

In the past, older adults were chronic victims of stigmatization or "ageism." Although ageism is dying a slow death, there remains a strong belief that older adults represent a homogeneous class when compared to younger groups. Relatedly, there remains a tendency to lump all older adults together in research and clinical studies. In actuality, nothing could be further from the truth. When normal individual variability as displayed in early life becomes augmented by the inherent differences in individual aging patterns, the result can be stated as a truism: *Variability (or Diversity) increases with age.* As a consequence, patterns of behavioral, mental, emotional and physiological function become more diverse and more difficult to predict solely on the basis of chronological age (Barry, 1977). This diversity has direct implications for the study of mental health issues of older adults. Fortunately, recent studies have attended to this rich diversity (e.g., Krause, Shaw, & Cairney, 2004).

There Are Limitations in Our Research

The field of gerontology has benefited immensely from the availability of longitudinal studies of aging (e.g., Nguyen & Zonderman, 2004; Shock et al., 1984). At the same time, much of our experimental data on aging patterns and behaviors has been derived from cross-sectional studies. In this well-known design, two or more different age groups are compared at one point in time across a specified dependent variable which might be reaction time, recognition memory, or level of depression. The results of such studies, though sometimes cited as evidence of aging decline and deterioration, actually provide information only relevant to *age differences* on the particular variable, and not *age changes* which can only be derived from longitudinal and time lag designs. Beyond the scope of this paper, the reader is referred to Birren and Schaie (2001) for information about research designs in aging research and the separation of the age, cohort and period effects. The important point is that the reader must exercise caution and a critical eye in reviewing studies addressing older adults' mental health issues.

It is also important to note that, until fairly recently, much of the mental health research on older adults was based upon institutionalized state hospital patients who typically displayed long histories of severe mental disorder and deteriorating conditions with continued hospitalization (Barry, 1977). Because of the well-known iatrogenic effects of long-term institutionalization (see Shorter, 1997), a highly distorted and pessimistic picture emerged which then portrayed older people as more helpless, dependent, and nonresponsive to therapeutic efforts. It is only within the last 25-35 years that a more accurate and optimistic picture of older adults' mental health has begun to emerge. This research is based upon healthier, active and noninstitionalized older adults who, incidentally, represent over 95% of our older population over 65 (e.g., see King, 2005).

Therapeutic Optimism Needs to Be the Norm

Related to the above, despite significant improvement in attitudes toward older adults and their potential for change, there continues to be a lingering degree of therapeutic pessimism that is reflected in the thinking of clinicians and researchers who work outside the field of gerontology and, to a lesser extent, for those working within the field. A somewhat greater pessimism continues to linger with respect to therapeutic efforts to help older adults who are experiencing cognitive impairment. These beliefs are a function of several factors, including past research that relied on institutionalized elderly, the antiquated view that mental health interventions for dementia patients were not helpful (see Malatesta, 1985), and the old view derived from traditional psychoanalytic thinking which posited that older adults were unsuitable candidates for psychoanalysis. The latter was interpreted by some to include mental health treatment in general. Fortunately, the situation has changed dramatically, and there is exciting research and clinical studies that are accumulating.

THE PLAN OF THE PROJECT

The ten manuscripts are organized according to the diagnostic classification system of the DSM-IV-TR (American Psychiatric Association, 2000). The project is divided into three sections. As sequenced in the

DSM-IV-TR, the first section contains three papers addressing mental disorders that possess either a primary neurological, brain-based etiology or are a function of substance abuse.

The first paper, by Peter Badgio, PhD, and Blaise Worden, MS, addresses the role of cognitive impairment in older women and men. This is an important topic that is relevant to all older adults, their families, caregivers, and treating health professionals. We are all concerned about our cognitive functioning, and many of us have offered a complaint now and then about how our memory has changed over the years. Dr. Badgio and Ms. Worden point out that "The challenge for the practitioner is to determine when such complaints signal the presence of a condition warranting further diagnostic assessment and treatment." In this regard, it is estimated that 50% or more of nursing home residents have a dementia diagnosis and that 34% of individuals residing in assisted living facilities have cognitive impairment (see Spira & Koven, 2005). Dr. Badgio and Ms. Worden cover the range of dementia types, and also include those that are a function of other medical conditions. An important section addresses cognitive impairment associated with conditions and treatments that are unique to women, including breast cancer treatment, menopause, and estrogen replacement therapy. Cognitive impairment associated with more controversial diagnoses is then addressed, along with cognitive difficulties related to emotional factors. Assessment and treatment guidelines are offered which emphasize the need for a multidisciplinary treatment plan that includes family members.

The second contribution, which addresses women, aging and alcohol use disorders is by Elizabeth Epstein, PhD, Kimberly Fischer-Elber, BA, and Zayed Al-Otaiba, MS. As the disparity between men's and women's drinking habits continues to decrease, the authors point out that the number and impact of older female drinkers is expected to increase dramatically over the next 20 years. Dr. Epstein and her colleagues note that women as they age are subject to an increasing physiological susceptibility to alcohol's effects, and that women of all ages are at higher risk for negative physical, social and psychological consequences associated with "at risk" and higher levels of alcohol consumption. An important section addresses barriers to detection and treatment of older women who display alcohol use problems. Finally, their discussion focuses on recommended assessment tools, in conjunction with a thorough review of treatment options, including more recent "elder-specific treatment programs."

Dr. Faith Dickerson, PhD, MPH, offers an important and sensitive presentation on older women who are suffering from schizophrenia–a serious and perhaps the most severe psychiatric disorder. Schizophrenia is typically a continuation of an illness first experienced during the younger adult years. It is noted that while about 67% of men and women go on to develop schizophrenia by the age of 40, the average age of onset for women is several years later and the majority of late onset cases are women. Dr. Dickerson also notes that older women, as other patients with schizophrenia, are vulnerable to substandard living conditions, poverty, and inadequate medical care. Moreover, it is pointed out that more typical problems of aging such as cognitive decline and chronic medical conditions may be exacerbated by schizophrenia. Offering a broad discussion of treatment approaches, including antipsychotic medications, Dr. Dickerson concludes by calling attention to the fact that older individuals with schizophrenia are disproportionately represented in boarding homes, adult foster care, and among the homeless.

The second section is composed of three presentations, including those addressing mood disorders, anxiety disorders, and post traumatic stress disorder. Focusing on major depressive disorder among older women, Reed Goldstein, PhD, and Alan Gruenberg, MD, offer a selective review of the psychiatric research on women, aging and major depressive disorder. They address a range of genetic, neurobiological and psychosocial studies. Although the reported rate of major depression in medically healthy older adults is less than that for younger cohorts, the rates increase significantly for older adults with co-morbid medical problems or other risk factors such as isolation. Moreover, depression in later life is associated with greater negative consequences, including functional decline, family stress, incomplete recovery, and higher rates of suicide (see Delano-Wood & Abeles, 2005). Late life mood disorders are also underdiagnosed and undertreated (see King, 2005). Drs. Goldstein and Gruenberg address special issues in the assessment and treatment of major depressive disorder in older adults, with a special focus on older women. Finally, they provide an informative discussion on related medical issues, pharmacotherapy, and psychotherapy approaches.

Stephen Levine, PhD, and Jay Weissman, PhD, in their comprehensive discussion of five major anxiety disorders, identify unique gender differences in the incidence and prevalence of anxiety disorders. Their section on etiological factors is thought-provoking and highlights the range of physical, mental and psychosocial factors that are associated with anxiety disorders in later life. Particularly informative is the section on how sensory changes in vision and hearing can contribute to development of anxiety, and on the role of incontinence in development of worry, anxiety and social avoidance. Drs. Levine and Weissman offer a discussion on therapeutic options that emphasize empirically supported treatments, including pharmacotherapy and behavioral and cognitive therapies.

The report on post traumatic stress disorder (PTSD) and older women is by Miriam Franco, MSW, PsyD. Her paper points out that women are more at risk for development of PTSD because of the high frequency of interpersonal trauma in the form of sexual abuse and domestic physical abuse. Older women are less likely to report traumatic symptoms and studies show that PTSD is underdiagnosed and misdiagnosed in older women. Recent research has shown a close relationship between trauma and health status among older adults (Krause et al., 2004), that dementia may intensify the effects of PTSD, and that age of childhood trauma may have persistent effects on the identity and personality of older adults (see Bernsten & Rubin, 2006). Finally, Dr. Franco's treatment section offers an eclectic blend of therapeutic approaches.

The third section includes presentations on dissociative disorders, sexual dysfunctions, eating disorders and borderline personality disorder. I felt that it would be important as well as prudent to include a presentation on a controversial DSM-IV-TR mental disorder that predominantly affects women, is under-recognized in older women, and is affected in various ways by the aging process. Dissociative identity disorder, formerly known as multiple personality disorder, is a complex and persistent response to severe childhood trauma that has been studied extensively by Richard Kluft, MD. While the reader may question and take issue with some of the concepts, he or she will nevertheless find it provocative, challenging and thought-provoking. Most importantly, Dr. Kluft provides a sensitive and realistic approach to managing complex dissociative disorders in older women.

With respect to sexual problems among older women, I had the unique opportunity to revisit a topic that I discussed 18 years ago in the *Journal of Women & Aging* (Malatesta, 1989). There have been several positive developments, including greater attention to the study of female sexuality, and recognition by the U.S. Surgeon General in 2001 that sexual health is connected with both physical and mental health, and that it is important throughout the entire life span. The development and popularization of Viagra, while benefiting many older men who might not have received treatment previously, has unwittingly reinforced an orgasm-oriented, functional approach to sexual activity that has extended to the pharmaceutical industry's attempt to find a female version of the drug. I address recent attempts to offer a more female focused diagnostic scheme for sexual problems that emphasizes the relationship, intimacy and a broad definition of sexuality. Finally, emphasis is placed on respecting the continuity of one's sexual lifestyle, and on a readiness to explore alternative methods of meeting the sexual needs of older women who are disabled, unpartnered, or living in a restricted environment.

Lynn Brandsma, PhD, offers an important and timely review of eating disorders in older women. Noting that while eating disorders have traditionally been viewed as disorders of adolescents and young women, recent research suggests that eating disorders often occur across the life span. Binge eating disorder may be particularly prevalent in middle aged and older women. Similarly, Dr. Brandsma focuses discussion on the issue of body image, and points out that insecurities about one's body can affect women of all ages, and can lead to eating disorder. Dr. Brandsma also reviews a range of adult developmental experiences that can trigger an eating disorder in middle aged and older women. She points out that an emerging clinical literature suggests that various lines of research are needed to explore and understand eating disorders among older women. Finally, Dr. Brandsma offers clinically useful guidelines for addressing eating disorder in older women.

One of the most complex and clinically challenging personality disorders, borderline personality disorder, is addressed by Melissa Hunt, PhD. While research on later life borderline conditions is limited, Dr. Hunt points out that some of their core features, including interpersonal difficulties, unstable mood and anger, remain relatively unchanged over time. In contrast, issues of impulsivity and identity disturbance tend to decline or are altered by the aging process. Dr. Hunt reviews etiological issues and addresses a range of effective treatment options, including pharmacotherapy, dialectical behavior therapy, schema focused cognitive therapy, and use of the therapeutic relationship. Finally, Dr. Hunt offers a fresh and innovative discussion regarding management of borderline personality disorder in the nursing home and other residential settings.

In closing this introduction, I trust that you will find the contributions to be informative, comprehensive and clinically useful. To the reader who is less familiar with the study of psychopathology, I hope that you will come away with the beginnings of a knowledge base from which to explore and study other aspects of mental health problems in older adults, and in older women in particular. For the clinician and counselor, I hope that the presentations are thought-provoking and illuminating, and that they complement your clinical work. At the same time, it is anticipated that the reader will gain an appreciation for areas of need and domains that should be addressed in future clinical and research studies. Obviously, there is much work to be done. We hope this project contributes to this process.

REFERENCES

Adams, H. E. (1981). *Abnormal psychology.* Dubuque, IA: Brown.

Adams, H. E., & Sutker, P. B. (Eds.) (2001). *Comprehensive handbook of Psychopathology* (3rd Edition). New York: Academic/Plenum.

American Psychiatric Association (2000). *DSM-IV-TR: Diagnostic and statistical manual of mental disorders* (4th Edition) Text Revision. Arlington, VA: American Psychiatric Association.

Barry, J. R. (1977). The psychology of aging. In J. R. Barry & C. R. Wingrove (Eds.), *Let's learn about aging: A book of readings.* New York: Halstead.

Bernsten, D., & Rubin, D. C. (2006). Flashbulb memories and posttraumatic stress reactions across the life span: Age-related effects of the German occupation of Denmark during World War II. *Psychology and Aging, 21,* 127-139.

Birren, J. E., & Schaie, K. W. (Eds.) (2001). *Handbook of the psychology of aging* (5th Edition). San Diego, CA: Academic Press.

Delano-Wood, L., & Abeles, N. (2005). Late-life depression: Detection, risk reduction, and somatic intervention. *Clinical Psychology: Science and Practice, 12,* 207-217.

Fisher, J. E., Zeiss, A. M., & Carstensen, L. L. (2001). Psychopathology in the aged. In H. E. Adams & P. B. Sutker (Eds.), *Comprehensive handbook of psychopathology* (3rd Edition) (pp. 921-951). New York: Academic/Plenum.

Gatz, M., & Smyer, M. (2001). Mental health and aging at the outset of the twenty-first century. In J. E. Birren & K. W. Shaie (Eds.), *Handbook of the psychology of aging* (5th Edition, pp. 523-544). San Diego, CA: Academic Press.

Hinrichsen, G. A. (2006). Why multicultural issues matter for practitioners working with older adults. *Professional Psychology: Research and Practice, 37,* 29-35.

Hobson, K. (2006). Hello, his and her healthcare. *U. S. News & World Report, 140* (8), 74-76.

Hughes, T. L., Smith, C., & Dan, A. (Eds.) (2003). *Mental health issues for sexual minority women.* Binghamton, NY: The Haworth Press, Inc.

King, D. A. (Ed.) (2005). Special issue: Assessment and treatment of depression in older adults. *Clinical Psychology: Science and Practice, 12,* 203-363.

Knight, B. G., Teri, L., Wohlford, P., & Santos. J. (Eds.) (1995). *Mental health services for older adults.* Washington, DC: American Psychological Association.

Krause, N., Shaw, B. A., & Cairney, J. (2004). A descriptive epidemiology of lifetime trauma and the physical health of older adults. *Psychology & Aging, 19,* 637-648.

Malatesta, V. J. (1985). Formulation of geriatric organic syndromes. In I. D. Turkat (Ed.), *Behavioral case formulation* (pp. 255-307). New York: Plenum Publishing.

Malatesta, V. J. (1989). Sexuality and the older adult: An overview with guidelines for the health care professional. *Journal of Women & Aging, 1*, 93-118.

Mickus, M., & Colenda, C. (2000). Knowledge of mental health benefits and provider preference. *Psychiatric Services, 51*, 199-203.

Nguyen, H. T., & Zonderman, A. B. (2006). Relationship between age and aspects of Depression: Consistency and reliability across two longitudinal studies. *Psychology and Aging, 21*, 119-126.

Shock, N. W., Greulich, R. C., Andres, R., Arenberg, D., Costa, P. et al. (1984). *Normal human aging: The Baltimore longitudinal study of aging* (NIH Publication No. 84-2450). Washington, DC: U. S. Government Printing Office.

Shorter, E. (1997). *A history of psychiatry: From the era of the asylum to the age of Prozac.* New York: Wiley & Sons.

Slater, L., Daniel, J. H., & Banks, A. E. (Eds.) (2003). *The complete guide to mental health for women.* Boston: Beacon Press.

Spira, A. P., & Koven, L. P. (2005). Long-term care: New challenges and opportunities for psychologists. *The Clinical Psychologist, 58*, 26-29.

Trotman, F. K., & C. Brody (Eds.) (2002). *Psychotherapy and counseling with older women.* New York: Springer.

U. S. Department of Health and Human Services (1999). *Mental health: A report by the Surgeon General.* Rockville, MD: Substance Abuse and Mental Health Services Administration, Center for Mental Health Services, National Institutes of Health, National Institute of Mental Health. Retrieved July 18, 2006, from http://www.surgeongeneral. gov/library/mentalhealth/home.html.

doi:10.1300/J074v19n01_01

Cognitive Functioning
and Aging in Women

Peter C. Badgio, PhD
Blaise L. Worden, MS

SUMMARY. Deficits in cognitive function may impact one's ability to attend to stimuli, think clearly, reason, and remember. Impaired cognitive function is a common complaint among older women presenting for treatment in both mental health and medical care settings, and differential diagnosis of type and extent of cognitive impairment is important for appropriate treatment planning and prognosis. Although overall gender differences in prevalence of cognitive dysfunction are minimal, it is important when treating older women to take into account unique challenges they face in the aging process that impact the cause, type and extent of cognitive complaints with which they present in clinical settings. The current paper provides an overview to guide accurate diagnosis, particularly in women, of different types of cognitive impairment under the broad category of dementias, including Alzheimer's, Lewy Body Disease, Vascular Dementia, and due to general medical conditions such as coronary artery bypass surgery, head injury, menopause, hypothyroidism, breast cancer treatment, Fibromyalgia, and chronic fatigue. In addition, emotional factors such as depression in older female patients complicate differential diagnosis of cognitive impairment and

---

Address correspondence to: Peter C. Badgio, 950 Haverford Road, Suite 305, Bryn Mawr, PA 19010 (E-mail: pbadgio@msn.com).

[Haworth co-indexing entry note]: "Cognitive Functioning and Aging in Women." Badgio, Peter C., and Blaise L. Worden. Co-published simultaneously in *Journal of Women & Aging* (The Haworth Press, Inc.) Vol. 19, No. 1/2, 2007, pp. 13-30; and: *Mental Health Issues of Older Women: A Comprehensive Review for Health Care Professionals* (ed: Victor J. Malatesta) The Haworth Press, Inc., 2007, pp. 13-30. Single or multiple copies of this article are available for a fee from The Haworth Document Delivery Service [1-800-HAWORTH, 9:00 a.m. - 5:00 p.m. (EST). E-mail address: docdelivery@haworthpress.com].

must be addressed. Given the multiplicity of causes of cognitive difficulties for women across the life span, careful assessment is crucial; the current paper reviews assessment strategies to prepare an integrated, biopsychosocial strategy for identifying particular cognitive deficits and related psychological and medical problems. In addition, prognostic indicators and treatment planning are discussed to help the practitioner organize an empathic, reasoned and multifaceted treatment approach to maximize recovery, minimize deterioration, and manage symptoms for older women in the context of their social support system and living environment. doi:10.1300/J074v19n01_02 *[Article copies available for a fee from The Haworth Document Delivery Service: 1-800-HAWORTH. E-mail address: <docdelivery@haworthpress.com> Website: <http://www.HaworthPress. com> © 2007 by The Haworth Press, Inc. All rights reserved.]*

KEYWORDS. Dementia, cognition, cognitive impairment, women, aging

Cognitive complaints such as "forgetfulness" are encountered frequently in both mental health and general medical practice settings. These complaints occur with increasing frequency with age. Women face unique challenges in assessment, differential diagnosis and treatment of conditions associated with impairment in cognitive functioning. The challenge for the practitioner is to pursue appropriate assessment of presenting problems in order to arrive at accurate diagnosis and prognosis, and offer therapy to patients and their families. In this paper, we describe the major causes of cognitive impairment, the different prevalence rates for the major causes of cognitive impairment in men and women, and describe causes of cognitive difficulties often encountered by women, or exclusively by women, as they progress through the aging process. The major features of the diagnostic entities associated with cognitive impairment are described, along with assessment techniques. Treatment issues, including the psychological and social needs of women with cognitive impairment, are identified.

DEMENTIAS

Cognitive functioning refers to mental functions such as attending, thinking, reasoning and memory. The dementias are the most commonly diagnosed condition in which cognitive deficits are the primary feature. The *Diagnostic and Statistical Manual of Mental Disorders–Fourth Edition, TR* (American Psychiatric Association, 2000) defines the diagnostic category *Dementia* as consisting of disorders that are characterized by memory impairment accompanied by one or more additional areas of cognitive deficit, due to the direct physiological effects of a general medical condition, the persisting effects of a substance, or multiple etiologies. The impairment in memory and at least one other cognitive domain must be severe enough to cause disruption in the individual's occupational or social functioning, and must represent a decline from a previously higher level of functioning.

Traditionally, the term dementia referred to conditions with a progressively deteriorating, irreversible course. The DSM-IV, however, has parted with the historical use of the term dementia, and now defines dementia on the basis of the pattern of cognitive deficits, rather than its longitudinal course. Thus, the term dementia now carries no connotation concerning future course or prognosis. A dementia may be progressive, or can have a static, or even remitting course, depending on the type of dementia. Types of dementia are distinguished based on etiology. For example, in dementia of the Alzheimer's type, the course is progressive and unremitting. In dementia caused by traumatic brain injury, the course is one of initial improvement, leading to full recovery or static plateau. The different types of dementia and their course are discussed below.

Diagnostically, dementia is to be distinguished from delirium and amnestic disorders. Memory impairment occurs in delirium and in amnestic disorders. In delirium, the cognitive deficits accompany a disturbance of consciousness. If memory impairment or other cognitive deficits occur only in the context of fluctuating delirium states, then a diagnosis of dementia is not offered. In some cases, a delirium can be superimposed on a dementia, in which cases both disorders are diagnosed, but there must be evidence of periods of cognitive deficit in the absence of delirium. Amnestic disorders are characterized by severe memory impairment. Amnestic disorders are distinguished from dementia in that in amnestic disorders, severe memory impairment occurs without other cognitive deficits, whereas in dementia, memory impairment must be accompanied by additional cognitive impairment.

There are other conditions in which cognitive complaints and deficits can be present, and presumed to be the result of the physiological effects of a known medical condition, but do not meet criteria for any of the specific dementias, amnestic disorders or deliriums. In some such cases, the cognitive difficulties are mild, or not a central focus in the overall clinical picture. In such cases, the preferred diagnosis is cognitive disorder not otherwise specified. Some of these conditions relevant to the subject of women and aging (e.g., cognitive complaints associated with menopause) will be discussed later in this article. Additionally, cognitive complaints also occur secondary to emotional disturbances such as depression. Particularly in the older adult, these conditions can sometimes be difficult to distinguish from some of the dementias. These conditions also will be discussed later in this article.

As indicated above, the presence of memory impairment is required to make a diagnosis of dementia and is a very prominent early symptom. Typical subjective complaints in early stages of a dementia include forgetting and/or repeating conversations, losing valuables, becoming lost and leaving food cooking on the stove. In late stages of a severe dementia, memory impairment can become so severe as to include previously acquired, familiar information such as an individual's own birthday, names of family members, occupation, and even one's own name. In addition to memory impairment, the diagnosis of dementia requires impairment in one or more additional areas, including language disturbance, apraxia, agnosia, and disturbance in executive functioning. Early forms of impaired language function typically include word finding difficulty and difficulty producing names. In more advanced stages, word finding difficulty in dementia can become increasingly severe such that the speech of such individuals becomes "empty," with reliance on vague references such as "thing" and "it." Comprehension of language can become impaired as well. Apraxia refers to impairment in the ability to execute motoric activities, despite intact basic motor and sensory functions. Such impairment can be manifest in difficulty dressing, drawing or using previously familiar appliances such as a coffee maker or sewing machine. Agnosia refers to the inability to recognize familiar objects, despite intact sensory function. A demented patient with agnosia can lose the ability to visually recognize familiar objects, such as a book or a pencil. Similarly, they can be unable to identify objects placed in their hands, despite intact tactile function. Executive mental functions refer to ability to plan, initiate, sequence and organize behavior. Executive mental deficits can be seen in difficulty completing novel tasks or even familiar tasks that involve multiple steps such as following a recipe, or doing laundry. Difficulties with multitasking or shifting from one task to another also represent impairment of executive function.

Dementia of the Alzheimer's Type

In Alzheimer's dementia, the course is characterized by a gradual, insidious onset and steady decline. Dementia of the Alzheimer's type is a diagnosis of exclusion, made after other central nervous system diseases, systemic conditions known to cause dementia and substance-induced conditions, are ruled out. The presence of a major psychiatric illness that could account for the cognitive symptoms such as a major depression must be ruled out as well. In making a diagnosis of dementia of the Alzheimer's type, one specifies subtype based on age of onset, with early onset referring to cases in which symptoms begin prior to the age of 65.

Prevalence rates for dementia of the Alzheimer's type vary across studies, depending in part on diagnostic criteria used. In all studies, prevalence increases with age beyond age 65, ranging from under 2% in the 65-69 year age range to approximately 20% over age 85. In general, most studies find that women are at somewhat higher risk for developing dementia of the Alzheimer's type. Andersen et al. (1999) report that based on a composite analysis of four studies including over 12,000 individuals ages 65 and over, women were at higher risk for developing Alzheimer's dementia, with an adjusted relative risk factor of 1.2. However, Ruitenberg et al. (2001) report that these gender differences emerge only at advanced age. In a large population-based perspective study of over 7,000 individuals 55 years and older, they found no gender difference in the incidence of Alzheimer's disease for age 90, but after age 90 the incidence was found to be higher for women than for men.

Lewy Body Disease

Dementia due to diffuse Lewy body disease is the second most common dementing illness, according to autopsy studies. It is more common than vascular dementia and is surpassed only by dementia of the Alzheimer's type (Beck, 1995; Stewart, 2003). Lewy body disease was identified in the mid 1980s, and its high incidence and clinical relevance have begun to be appreciated only recently. Lewy bodies refer to the neuronal bodies seen in the mid brains of patients suffering from Parkinson's disease. In patients suffering from Lewy body dementia, they are spread more diffusely and are seen throughout the cortex (Kalra, Bergeron, & Lang, 1996).

Clinically, diffuse Lewy body dementia shares features with both Alzheimer's disease and Parkinson's disease. The cognitive deficits seen in Lewy body disease are similar to those found in Alzheimer's disease, yet in Lewy body disease the symptoms generally vary a great deal from one day to the next, whereas day-to-day variability in Alzheimer's disease is much less marked. Mild to moderate parkinsonian symptoms start generally at the same time as the cognitive impairment in Lewy body disease. Lewy body disease is distinguished by the high incidence of psychotic symptoms, including purely visual hallucinations (the most common psychotic symptom). Further, in diffuse Lewy body disease, psychotic symptoms are much more prominent and occur much earlier in the course of illness than is the case with Alzheimer's dementia (Ballard et al., 1999). Interestingly, these symptoms often are not distressing to the patients who have them. It is crucial to note that patients with diffuse Lewy body dementia can have severe, adverse reactions to antipsychotic medications (Ballard et al., 1998). Thus, accurate, early diagnosis is critical.

Dementia due to diffuse Lewy body disease is almost twice as common in men as in women. Nevertheless, it is a common form of dementia, accounting for 15-20% of all dementias, and therefore warrants clinical consideration by those treating women.

Vascular Dementia

Vascular dementia (or multi-infarct dementia), the third most common type of dementia, also is more common among men than women in all age groups (American Psychiatric Association, 2001; Ruitenberg, 2001). In contrast to dementia of the Alzheimer's type, which has a slow and insidious onset, the onset of vascular dementia typically is abrupt and has a stepwise, fluctuating course rather than a slow and steady progression. The course is quite variable across individuals. Diagnostically, the presence of memory impairment and impairment in one or more other areas of cognitive functioning is required, as with other dementias. In addition, a diagnosis of vascular dementia requires focal neurological signs and symptoms (such as sensory and/or motor findings upon neurological exam), as well as laboratory evidence of cerebrovascular disease.

Dementias and Cognitive Disorders Due to General Medical Conditions

While the vast majority of dementias are due to Alzheimer's disease, diffuse Lewy body disease, and cerebrovascular disease, there are numerous other medical conditions that can produce cognitive impairment of sufficient pervasiveness and severity to warrant a diagnosis of dementia. When there is evidence from the history, physical examination, or laboratory findings that a medical condition is present that is causally related to the dementia, the appropriate diagnosis is dementia due to that specific condition. When the cognitive impairment associated with a general medical condition is not of the pervasiveness and severity to warrant a diagnosis of dementia, but nevertheless clinically significant and of concern to the patient, the appropriate diagnosis is Cognitive Disorder Not Otherwise Specified (NOS). The medical conditions that can produce dementias or cognitive disorders are too numerous to cover here. In this paper, we cover several conditions that are relevant to women's health and aging, but this should not be considered an exhaustive discussion of all conditions in which cognitive impairment can be a prominent feature.

Coronary artery bypass surgery. Coronary-artery bypass grafting surgery results in a rather high prevalence of cognitive decline. Newman et al. (2001) found that 53% of patients at discharge exhibited cognitive decline. While many patients exhibited a pattern of early improvement, early improvement often was followed by later decline. There are no data on differential risk of cognitive decline in men versus women. Further, there is no agreed upon mechanism for the observed cognitive impairment.

Head injury. Typically, head injury is considered a young persons' health issue, and young males' health issue at that. Traumatic brain injuries in the population are most common among adult males ages 16-25. What is less well appreciated, is that older adults are a high risk group as well (Fields & Coffey, 1994). Following a period of relatively low risk in the middle adult years, adults are at increased risk for traumatic brain injury once they reach an age of 65-70. In addition, older adults are more vulnerable to the development of post-injury complications, such as subdural hematoma and intracranial hemorrhage. Moreover, the large sex difference that is evident in the younger years when men are at higher risk disappears in the later years, at which point women are at an equally high risk as men (Sorenson & Kraus, 1991).

Falls are the most frequent cause of head injuries among older adults. There are various symptoms and medical conditions that occur with increasing frequency as individuals age that are associated with increased risk for falling, such as dizziness, visual disturbance, motor impairment, decreased reaction time, etc. Among older women, falls often occur in the home, and might not be witnessed or brought to medical attention. Thus, increased awareness of the possible occurrence and likely sequelae of traumatic brain injury among older women is warranted for those working with this population.

The cognitive consequences of traumatic brain injury include impairment in memory, attention, concentration, mental processing speed and possibly other cognitive functions. The vast majority of traumatic brain injuries (80% or greater) are mild injuries, characterized by brief or no loss of consciousness at the time of the injury. In cases of mild traumatic brain injury without further complications, even among older individuals, these impairments should recover over a period of weeks and months following the injury. Older adults have long been thought to have a more difficult course of recovery following traumatic brain injury than younger adults. This is more likely to be true for moderate and severe injuries. Regardless of severity, barring post-injury complications, the post-injury course is one of improvement reaching full recovery or plateau, rather than progressive decline. In cases where there is an apparent decline, or in which cognitive complaints persist longer than would be expected based on the nature of the injury, other complicating factors must be considered. Particularly in an aging population, preexisting and comorbid conditions affecting cognitive functioning often are present that can be misattributed to the head injury.

Menopause. Complaints of cognitive decline during menopause are often secondary to more salient symptom presentations such as fatigue, irritability, and vasomotor symptoms (i.e., hot flashes). Nevertheless, a significant number of women experience cognitive decline as they pass through menopause, and complaints of memory difficulties are frequent in primary care settings. In one study, 44.4% of 4,158 early and late perimenopausal women endorsed "forgetfulness" on a self-report of current symptoms, as compared with the 31% of premenopausal women (Gold et al., 2000). In another sample of 230 women (randomly selected from census information on race and income) with a mean age of 46.7 (*SD* = 4.4), 62% reported undesirable memory changes over the few years prior to their interview (Mitchell & Woods, 2001). In particular, these women complained about increasing difficulty in recall of words and numbers. However, many women do not link changes in cognitive ability to their menopausal state (O'Connell, 2005) and often attribute changes in cognition to aging (Mitchell & Woods, 2001).

Given that many women fail to connect symptoms to the menopausal stage, study outcomes based on self-reports of cognitive changes during and after menopause might be inaccurate. It is preferable to examine studies using reliable neuropsychological testing of cognitive function. There are several neuropsychological tests on which menopausal and postmenopausal women show cognitive deficiencies. Meyer et al. (2003) administered the Digit Span Backward (DSB) subtest and the

Symbol Digit Modality Test (SDMT) from the Wechsler Memory Scale to 771 women in the menopausal transition. They found a slight increase over time in scores on the DSB subtest, but found a decrease in cognitive performance on the SDMT task in postmenopausal women. It has also been found that menopausal women not treated with estrogen therapy made more preservative errors on the California Verbal Learning Test (CVLT), which is a test of retention of information and semantic recall (Keenan, Ezzat, Ginsburg, & Moore, 2001). This study also found that untreated women had significantly worse performance on a test of working memory. Finally, levels of circulating estrogen in elderly women have been found to be correlated with better delayed verbal recall negatively on the Wechsler Memory Scale (Drake et al., 2000).

The body of literature on hormone replacement therapy (HRT) and its effects on cognitive functioning is substantial, and a full discussion would go far beyond the scope of this paper. Findings have been highly inconsistent, depending in part on sample characteristics, the cognitive tests used and HRT dosage, but most studies have found HRT-related cognitive benefits on at least some cognitive tests (Dunkin et al., 2005; Zec & Trivedi, 2002). A finding that has been most consistent across studies is HRT's effect of maintaining or enhancing verbal memory abilities (Fluck, File, & Rymer, 2002; Sherwin, 1996).

Much has been written on the question of whether or not hormone replacement therapy benefits cognition in older women generally, and whether hormone replacement therapy has specific, beneficial effects in reducing the risk of or reducing symptoms of Alzheimer's disease. Until recently, there had been hope that hormone replacement therapy could help avert cognitive decline in aging women. Some epidemiological studies supported this notion. In a study of 2,073 non-demented women over the age of 65, postmenopausal HRT was associated with better global cognition and reduced decline (Carlson et al., 2001). Other large-scale epidemiological studies, however, failed to reveal a relationship between HRT and cognitive performance among older women (Kang et al., 2004).

The Women's Health Initiative (WHI) represents the largest, double blind, clinical trial study involving hormone replacement therapy. WHI data fail to reveal significant benefits of HRT on global cognitive functioning as assessed by the Mini Mental Status Exam (Hays et al., 2003), or memory tasks (Rapp et al., 2003; Espeland et al., 2004). Additionally, other health risks have been associated with long-term HRT.

Hypothyroidism. For women over the age of 65, the incidence of hypothyroidism has been estimated to be between 5-15%. Hypothyroidism is associated with cognitive deficits, including reduced information processing speed, slowness to respond to questions and memory retrieval deficits. Many of the cognitive and physical symptoms of hypothyroidism resemble changes that accompany normal aging. Moreover, symptoms of hypothyroidism might be less pronounced or noticeable when the condition has a gradual onset. Therefore, hypothyroidism often goes undetected. Hypothyroidism is an important diagnostic consideration in cases of older women with cognitive complaints, as the symptoms can be reversible with appropriate treatment (Burmeister et al., 2001).

Breast cancer treatments. Breast cancer is the most common form of malignancy among women in the United States. Adjuvant chemotherapy and hormone suppression (tamoxifen) have improved treatment response (Bender et al., 2001). Women receiving adjuvant chemotherapy alone or with tamoxifen frequently complain of impaired cognitive function. Several studies have demonstrated impaired cognitive test performance associated with these breast cancer treatments. Brezden et al. (2000) compared women receiving adjuvant chemotherapy post-breast cancer surgery to women who received breast cancer surgery alone and found poorer cognitive functioning scores among patients receiving adjuvant therapy. The anti-estrogen therapy, tamoxifen, in addition to standard chemotherapy or alone also has been associated with cognitive deficits. Jenkins et al. (2003) found specific deficits on measures of processing speed and verbal memory among women receiving tamoxifen therapy for treatment of breast cancer. In a study using standardized neuropsychological test instruments, Castellon et al. (2004) compared women who received adjuvant chemotherapy alone or in conjunction with tamoxifen following breast cancer surgery with those who received only breast cancer surgery. They report that patients who received adjuvant chemotherapy in addition to breast cancer surgery performed significantly worse on tests of verbal learning, visuospatial functioning and visual memory than those receiving breast cancer surgery alone. Those who received both chemotherapy and tamoxifen showed the greatest impairment.

Notably, the Castellon et al. study found that there was no relationship between patients' subjective complaints of cognitive impairment and their objective test performance. Instead, subjective complaints of cognitive difficulty were associated with measures of fatigue and emotional distress, but not objectively measured functioning. This finding points to the importance of careful, objective assessment of cognitive ability in women with cognitive complaints, as discussed below.

Fibromyalgia. Fibromyalgia is a common diagnosis among patients presenting with chronic musculoskeletal pain. The etiology of the pain is not known and the diagnosis remains somewhat controversial. The role of organic illness has been questioned and some have considered the condition to be psychogenic or psychosomatic in nature. Nevertheless, the diagnosis has increasingly been accepted and is considered the most common condition of generalized musculoskeletal pain in women between the ages of 20-55 years. Fibromyalgia is 10 times more common in women than men. Among women, the prevalence increases from approximately 2% at age 20 to 8% at age 70 (Goldenberg, 1987, 2005). Fatigue is present in the majority of cases in which fibromyalgia is diagnosed. Complaints of impaired cognitive function are common in fibromyalgia, particularly short-term memory loss. In a study comparing non-depressed fibromyalgia patients with age matched controls (Park et al., 2001), fibromyalgia patients performed more poorly than age matched controls on numerous measures of memory, recall and verbal fluency, but not on measures of processing speed.

Chronic fatigue. Like fibromyalgia, chronic fatigue syndrome is a complicated and somewhat controversial diagnosis. Diagnostic criteria vary and overlap considerably with fibromyalgia. The central feature is unexplained fatigue. Typical diagnostic criteria such as that offered by the Centers for Disease Control require additional associated symptoms. Only a subset of patients with complaints of chronic fatigue meet diagnostic criteria for chronic fatigue syndrome. Most studies employing common diagnostic criteria find chronic fatigue syndrome to be about twice as common in women. Many possible etiologies have been posited, including infectious diseases (Gluckman, 2005).

Patients with chronic fatigue syndrome commonly complain of impaired cognitive function, including difficulties with concentration, attention and memory. Objective studies of cognitive test performance among persons with chronic fatigue syndrome have yielded variable results. Moreover, individual patients' performance has been found to vary considerably across time and across tasks (Fuentes et al., 2001). Chronic fatigue patients have been found to underestimate the quality of their own cognitive functioning (Metzger & Denney, 2002). Importantly, patients' perceptions of their own conditions and causes of their perceived difficulties significantly affect the quality of their cognitive functioning and performance. Smith and Sullivan (2003) examined the cognitive test performance among chronic fatigue syndrome patients who perceive their conditions to be adversely affected by chemical exposure. In a double blind, placebo controlled study, they examined patients' perceptions and test performance following exposure to chemical substances or placebo. Cognitive test performance was affected by patients' subjective perception of whether they had been exposed to a chemical substance, but not by whether they were actually exposed to a chemical substance or placebo. Thus, patients' beliefs and expectations regarding their cognitive functioning affected their objective performance.

Whatever the underlying cause(s) of chronic fatigue syndrome, comorbid depression, anxiety and other psychological difficulties are very common in chronic fatigue syndrome. Although chronic fatigue syndrome and perceived disability tend to be chronic, psychiatric status has been found to be predictive of improvement in subjective well-being and in cognitive performance (Tiersky et al., 2001) among patients with the diagnosis.

EMOTIONAL FACTORS

As noted above in conditions such as traumatic brain injury and chronic fatigue syndrome, emotional factors and patients' expectations strongly influence both their subjective cognitive complaints and their actual cognitive test performance. For example, O'Boyle et al. (1990) found that among elderly depressed patients as well as non-depressed individuals, subjective cognitive complaints were not related to actual scores on objective assessment of cognitive functioning, but highly correlated with depressive symptoms. Depression is significantly more prevalent among women than men. Thus, assessment for the presence of depressive and other emotional symptoms is an important diagnostic consideration for older women presenting with cognitive complaints.

The older adult presenting with cognitive complaints and depression remains one of the more difficult differential diagnostic problems facing health-care professionals. One must determine whether cognitive problems are secondary to the mood disorder, represent a dementia or other medical condition, or some combination. For example, there is considerable symptom overlap in major depression and dementia of the Alzheimer's type. Symptoms such as apathy, sleep difficulty, personality change, and agitation are typical of Alzheimer's, but can also represent a mood disorder (Kaszniak & Christenson, 1994). While subjective complaints and manifest symptoms in primary dementias and depressive disorders overlap greatly, particularly at mild to moderate levels of severity, detailed evaluation, history, and clinical course can help differentiate the two types of conditions. Determining the onset of mood symptoms relative to onset of cognitive symptoms helps to determine which condition is primary; however, patients often are unable to recollect this history, and involvement of close family members in the assessment might be necessary. Additionally, the pattern of test scores observed on comprehensive neuropsychological evaluation can differentiate between mood disorders and primary dementias. Similarly, brain imaging studies provide further data. No single source of data can determine the differential diagnosis and distinguish primary cognitive deficits from the effects of emotional factors, underscoring the importance of comprehensive and multidisciplinary evaluation of older women with emotional and cognitive symptoms.

ASSESSMENT AND TREATMENT CONSIDERATIONS

Given the multiplicity of causes of cognitive difficulties in women across the life span, careful assessment and accurate diagnosis are crucial. Some causes of cognitive impairment are treatable and even reversible such as emotional disturbance and hormonal imbalance, thus making accurate diagnosis essential for good outcome. Even in non-reversible cases, accurate diagnosis is important in designing treatments to slow the progression and/or minimize the negative impact of symptoms, as well as providing useful information regarding prognosis and course of illness to patients and their families.

Assessment is a multifaceted undertaking that should follow a biopsychosocial model, involving medical, psychological, and family input in the overall evaluation. A thorough physical exam, medical history and review of medications are instrumental in identifying many causes of cognitive impairment. More specialized and technological assessments such as brain imaging studies often are required. Attention also must be given to alcohol and other substance use or possible abuse (see Epstein et al., this volume). Detailed assessments of cognitive functioning and other psychological factors also form part of the diagnostic work-up. Identification of emotional factors such as depression often can be made with a skilled interview and history. In unclear or complex cases, formal psychometric testing by a psychologist is indicated. As subjective cognitive complaints often are not correlated with actual cognitive ability for a variety of reasons, objective assessment of mental status is a necessary component of assessing the patient with cognitive complaints in general medical and psychological settings. The Mini Mental Status Exam (Teng & Chui, 1987) is the most widely utilized, brief assessment instrument. It is a scored, brief assessment of a broad range of cognitive functions that can be administered by trained health-care staff. Scored, objective instruments such as the Mini Mental Status Exam can be administered longitudinally to track changes in cognitive function, including treatment response.

A comprehensive neuropsychological evaluation is a highly valuable piece of the assessment and treatment process. The pattern of deficits across different domains of cognitive functioning can help determine the underlying cause of impairment and thus aid in differential diagnosis. Neuropsychological testing also can identify preserved cognitive strengths that can be utilized to help patients compensate for impaired areas of function, and to pursue enriching activities that provide continuing quality of life.

Involvement of close family members can prove invaluable in assessing the nature and possible causes of cognitive impairment. Those living with the patient can help to provide a history regarding the onset and progression of symptoms, as well as the quality of functioning in the home environment. Assessment of family also helps to identify needs to help the woman with cognitive impairment adapt to changes in her functioning within the home environment. For example, women who have occupied the role of caretaker within the home often have difficulty adapting to the new role of needing to accept care from others, and other family members also need help adapting to such role changes.

Clear and comprehensive feedback to patients and their families is a crucial first step in treatment. Counseling patients and their families regarding the nature and expected course of their conditions is itself therapeutic and part of the overall treatment and management of women with cognitive deficits. For example, in cases of progressively deteriorating dementias, early detection and diagnosis allow patients to participate in decision making regarding the expected future changes in their lives. Additionally, patients' expectations and physician response have been shown to contribute to outcome and perceived recovery in conditions such as brain injury (Putnam et al., 1996). Thus, providing patients with appropriate, realistic explanations and expectations can facilitate natural recovery, whereas excessive focus on symptoms and/or misattribution of subjective complaints to an injury can lead to a protracted period of perceived disability.

In cases of moderate to severe dementing illness, careful management of the patient's environment to ensure safety and predictability is indicated. Home safety around functions such as cooking must be assessed. Likewise, driving safety is an issue to be raised and driving safety evaluations are available in most major rehabilitation settings. Often, a move to a simpler, more structured environment with available continuum of care as the illness progresses is a necessary step in the care of the older woman with cognitive impairment. Such a move is a stressful time in the lives of women and their families, but if handled well, can facilitate their overall adaptation and quality of life. In addition to safety in the physical environment, the social environment and activity of patients with cognitive impairment comprise aspects of a comprehensive approach to treatment. A socially supportive and safe environment, with a range of activities that do not create frustration, comprises the most effective, long-term treatment for primary, degenerative dementia (Nixon, 1996). In addition to care of the patient, support for family, caregivers and close friends is part of treatment.

As patients with progressive dementias or medical conditions causing cognitive impairment negotiate the complicated health-care system, with numerous specialists and diagnostic workups, along with other life changes that these conditions often necessitate, it is the trusted mental health professional or primary health-care provider who can offer the greatest consistency and comfort as a trusted helping professional and source of reliable information. Therefore, knowledge of these conditions and the ability to recognize, assess and monitor them enhances good clinical practice.

REFERENCES

American Psychiatric Association (2000). *Diagnostic and statistical manual of mental disorders, text revision* (4th ed.). Washington, DC.

Andersen, K., Launer, L.J., Dewey, M.E. et al. (1999). Gender differences in the incidence of AD and vascular dementia. The EURODEM studies. *Neurology, 53* (Dec.), 1992-1997.

Angelopoulos, N., Barbounis, V., Livadas, S., Kaltsas, D., & Tolis, G. (2004). Effects of estrogen deprivation due to breast cancer treatment. *Endocrine-Related Cancer, 11*(3), 523-535.

Ballard, C., Grace, J., McKeith, I. et al. (1998). Neuroleptic sensitivity in dementia with Lewy bodies and Alzheimer's disease. *Lancet, 351* (9108), 1032-1033.

Ballard, C., Holmes, C., McKeith, I. et al. (1999). Psychiatric morbidity in dementia with Lewy bodies: A prospective clinical and neuropathological comparative study with Alzheimer's disease. *American Journal of Psychiatry, 156*(7), 1039-1045.

Beck, B.J. (1995). Neuropsychiatric manifestations of diffuse Lewy body disease. *Journal of Geriatric Psychiatry and Neurology, 8*(3), 189-196.

Bender, C.M., Paraska, K.K., Sereika, S.M., Ryan, C.M., & Berga, S.L. (2001). Cognitive function and reproductive hormones in adjuvant therapy for breast cancer: A critical review. *Journal of Pain and Symptom Management, 21*(5), 407-424.

Brezden, C.B., Phillips, K., Abdolell, M., Bunston, T., & Tannock, I.F. (2000). Cognitive function in breast cancer patients receiving adjuvant chemotherapy. *Journal of Clinical Oncology, 18*(14), 2695-2701.

Burmeister, L.A., Ganguli, M., Dodge, H.H. et al. (2001). Hypothyroidism and cognition: Preliminary evidence for a specific defect in memory. *Thyroid, 11*, 1177.

Carlson, M.C., Zandi, P.P., Plassman, B.L. et al. (2001). Hormone replacement therapy and reduced cognitive decline in older women: The Cache County Study. *Neurology, 57*, 2210-2216.

Castellon, S.A., Ganz, P.A., Bower, J.E., Petersen, L., Abraham, L., & Greendale, G.A. (2004). Neurocognitive performance in breast cancer survivors exposed to adjuvant chemotherapy and Tamoxifen. *Journal of Clinical and Experimental Neuropsychology, 26*(7), 955-969.

Drake E.B., Henderson V.W., Stanczyk, F.Z., McCleary, C.A., Brown W.S., Smith C.A., Rizzo A.A., Murdock, G.A., & Buckwalter, J.G. (2000). Associations between circulating sex steroid hormones and cognition in normal elderly women. *Neurology, 54*(3), 599-603.

Dunkin, J., Rasgon, N., Wagner-Steh, K., David, S., Altshuler, L., & Rapkin, A. (2005). Reproductive events modify the effects of estrogen replacement therapy on cognition in healthy postmenopausal women. *Psychoneuroendocrinology, 30*(3), 284-296.

Epstein, E.E., Fischer-Elber, K., & Al-Otaiba, Z. Women, aging, and alcohol use disorders. (This volume)

Espeland, M.A., Rapp, S.R., Shumaker, S.A., Brunner, R., Manson, J.E., Sherwin, B.B. et al. (2004). Conjugated equine estrogens and global cognitive function in postmenopausal women. *Journal of the American Medical Association, 291*, 2959-2968.

Fields, R.B., & Coffey, C.E. (1994). Traumatic brain injury. In C.E. Coffey, J.L. Cummings, M.R. Lovell, & G.D. Pearlson (Eds.), *The American Psychiatric Press textbook of geriatric neuropsychiatry* (pp. 479-507). Washington, DC: American Psychiatric Association.

Fluck, E., File, S.E., & Rymer, J. (2002). Cognitive effects of 10 years of hormone-replacement therapy with tibolone. *Journal of Clinical Psychopharmacology, 22*(1), 62-67.

Fuentes, K., Hunter, M.A., Strauss, S., & Hultsch, D.F. (2001). Intra-individual variability in cognitive performance in persons with chronic fatigue syndrome. *The Clinical Neuropsychologist, 15*(2), 210-227.

Gluckman, S.J. (2005). Clinical features and diagnosis of chronic fatigue syndrome. Retrieved December 14, 2005 from www.uptodate.com.

Gold, E.B., Sternfeld, B., Kelsey, J.L., Brown, C., Mouton, C., Reame, N., Salamone, L., & Stellato, R. (2000). Relation of demographic and lifestyle factors to symptoms in a multi-racial/ethnic population of women 40-55 years of age. *American Journal of Epidemiology, 152*(5), 463-473.

Goldenberg, D.L. (2005). Clinical manifestations and diagnosis of fibromyalgia in adults. Retrieved December 13, 2005 from www.uptodate.com.

Goldenberg, D.L. (1987). Fibromyalgia syndrome: An emerging but controversial condition. *JAMA, 257,* 2782.

Hays, J., Ockene, J.K., Brunner, R.L., Kotchen, J.M., Manson, J.E., Patterson, R.E. et al. (2003). Effects of estrogen plus progestin on health-related quality of life. *New England Journal of Medicine, 348,* 1839-1854.

Jenkins, V., Shilling, V., Fallowfield, L., Howell, A., & Hutton, S. (2003). Does hormone therapy for the treatment of breast cancer have a detrimental effect on memory and cognition? A pilot study. *Psycho-Oncology, 13,* 61-66.

Kalra, S., Bergeron, C., & Lang, A.E. (1996). Lewy body disease and dementia: A review. *Archives of Internal Medicine, 156*(5), 487-493.

Kang, J.H., Weuve, J., & Grodstein, F. (2004). Postmenopausal hormone therapy and risk of cognitive decline in community-dwelling aging women. *Neurology, 63,* 101.

Kaszniak, A.W., & Christenson, G.D. (1994). Differential diagnosis of depression and dementia. In M. Storandt & G.R. VandenBos (Eds.), *Neuropsychological assessment of dementia and depression in older adults: A clinical guide.* Washington, DC: The American Psychological Association.

Keenan, P.A., Ezzat, W.H., Ginsburg, K., & Moore G.J. (2001). Prefrontal cortex as the site of estrogen's effect on cognition. *Psychoneuroendocrinology, 26*(6), 577-590.

Kosaka, K., Yoshimura, M., Ikeda, K. et al. (1984). Diffuse type of Lewy body disease: Progressive dementia with abundant cortical Lewy bodies and senile changes of varying degree–a new disease? *Clinical Neuropathology, 3*(5), 185-192.

Kritz-Silverstein, D., & Barrett-Connor, E. (2002). Hysterectomy, oophorectomy, and cognitive function in older women. *Journal of the American Geriatrics Society, 50* (1), 55-61.

Metzger, F.A., & Denney, D.R. (2002). Perception of cognitive performance in patients with chronic fatigue syndrome. *Annals of Behavioral Medicine, 24*(2), 106-112.

Meyer, P.M., Powell, L.H., Wilson, R.S., Everson-Rose, S.A., Kravitz, H.M., Luborsky, J.L., Madden, T., Pandey, D., & Evans, D.A. (2003). A population-based longitudinal study of cognitive functioning in the menopausal transition. *Neurology, 61*(6), 801-806.

Morse, C.A., & Rice, K. (2005). Memory after menopause: Preliminary considerations of hormone influence on cognitive functioning. *Archives of Women's Mental Health, 8*(3), 155-162.

Newman, M.F., Kirchner, J.L., Phillips-Bute, B., Gaver, V., Grocott, H., Jones, R.H. et al. (2001). Longitudinal assessment of neurocognitive function after coronary-artery bypass surgery. *The New England Journal of Medicine, 344*(6), 395-402.

Nixon, S.J. (1996). Alzheimer's disease and vascular dementia. In R.L. Adams, O.A. Parsons, J.L. Culbertson, & S.J. Nixon (Eds.), *Neuropsychology for clinical practice: Etiology, assessment, and treatment of common neurological disorders.* Washington, DC: American Psychological Association.

O'Boyle, M., Amadeo, M., & Self, D. (1990). Cognitive complaints in elderly depressed and pseudodemented patients. *Psychology and Aging, 5*(3), 467-468.

O'Connell, E. (2005). Mood, energy, cognition, and physical complaints: A mind/body approach to symptom management during the climacteric. *Journal of Obstetric, Gynecologic, & Neonatal Nursing, 34*(2), 274-279.

Park, D.C., Glass, J.M., Minear, M., & Crafford, L.J. (2001). Cognitive function in fibromyalgia patients. *Arthritis & Rheumatism, 44*(9), 2125-2133.

Putnam, S.H., Millis, S.R., & Adams, K.M. (1996). Mild traumatic brain injury: Beyond cognitive assessment. In I. Grant & K.M. Adams (Eds.), *Neuropsychological assessment of neurological disorders* (2nd ed.). New York: Oxford University Press.

Rapp, S.R., Espeland, M.A., Shumaker, S.A., Henderson, V.W., Brunner, R.L., Manson, J.E. et al. (2003). Effect of estrogen plus progestin on global cognitive function in postmenopausal women. Women's Health Initiative Memory Study: A randomized controlled trial. *Journal of the American Medical Association, 289*, 2663-72.

Ruitenberg, A., Ott, A., van Swieten, J.C., Hofman, A., & Breteler, M.M.B. (2001). Incidence of dementia: Does gender make a difference? *Neurobiology of Aging, 22*, 575-580.

Sherwin, B.B. (2005). Estrogen and memory in women: How can we reconcile the findings? *Hormones & Behavior, 47*(3), 371-375.

Sherwin, B.B. (1996). Hormones, mood, and cognitive functioning in postmenopausal women. *Obstetrics & Gynecology, 87*(2), 20S-26S.

Smith, S., & Sullivan, K. (2003). Examining the influence of biological and psychological factors on cognitive performance in chronic fatigue syndrome: A randomized, double-blind, placebo-controlled, crossover study. *International Journal of Behavioral Medicine, 10*(2), 106-173.

Sorenson, S.B., & Kraus, J.F. (1991). Occurrence, severity, and outcomes of brain injury. *Journal of Head Trauma Rehabilitation, 6*(2), 1-10.

Stewart, J.T. (2003). Defining diffuse Lewy body disease. Postgraduate Medicine On Line. 113 (5). Retrieved 11/21/2005 from www.postgradmed.com/issues/2003/05_03/stewart2.htm.

Sullivan, M.E., & Fugate-Woods, N. (2001). Midlife women's attributions about perceived memory changes: Observations from the Seattle Midlife Women's Health Study. *Journal of Women's Health & Gender-Based Medicine, 10*(4), 351-362.

Teng, E.L., & Chui, H.C. (1987). The Modified Mini-Mental State (3MS) Examination. *Journal of Clinical Psychology, 48*(8), 314-318.

Tiersky, L.A., DeLuca, J., Hill, N., Dhar, S.K., Johnson, S.K., Lange, G., Rappolt, G., & Natelson, B.H. (2001). Longitudinal assessment of neuropsychological functioning, psychiatric status, functional disability and employment status in chronic fatigue syndrome. *Applied Neuropsychology, 8*(1), 41-50.

Zandi, P.P., Carlson, M.C., Plassman, B.L., Welsh-Bohmer, K.A., Mayer, L.S., Steffens, D.C., & Breitner, J.C. (2002). Hormone replacement therapy and incidence of Alzheimer disease in older women: The Cache County Study. *JAMA: Journal of the American Medical Association, 288*(17), 2123-2129.

Zec, R.F., & Trivedi, M.A. (2002). The effects of estrogen replacement therapy on neuropsychological functioning in postmenopausal women with and without dementia: A critical and theoretical review. *Neuropsychology Review, 12*(2), 65-109.

doi:10.1300/J074v19n01_02

Women, Aging, and Alcohol Use Disorders

Elizabeth E. Epstein, PhD
Kimberly Fischer-Elber, BA
Zayed Al-Otaiba, MS

SUMMARY. The increase in prevalence rates of alcohol use disorders in younger versus older cohorts of female drinkers is many times higher than the corresponding increase in prevalence rates for male drinkers. Thus, the number and impact of older female drinkers is expected to increase over the next 20 years as the disparity between men's and women's drinking rates decrease. Due to differences in metabolism of alcohol, women of all ages compared to men are at higher risk for negative physical, medical, social, and psychological consequences associated with at-risk and higher levels of alcohol consumption. Aging women face new sets of antecedents related to challenges in the middle and older adult phases of life, such as menopause, retirement, "empty nest," limited mobility, and illness. As women age, they are subject to an even greater physiological susceptibility to alcohol's effect, as well as to a risk of synergistic effects of alcohol in combination with prescription drugs. On the other hand, there is mixed research indicating that older women may benefit from the buffering effect of low levels of alcohol on hormonal declines associated with menopause, perhaps serving as a pro-

---

Address correspondence to: Elizabeth E. Epstein, Center of Alcohol Studies, 607 Allison Road, Rutgers–The State University of New Jersey, Piscataway, NJ 08854 (E-mail: bepstein@rci.rutgers.edu).

[Haworth co-indexing entry note]: "Women, Aging, and Alcohol Use Disorders." Epstein, Elizabeth E., Kimberly Fischer-Elber, and Zayed Al-Otaiba. Co-published simultaneously in *Journal of Women & Aging* (The Haworth Press, Inc.) Vol. 19, No. 1/2, 2007, pp. 31-48; and: *Mental Health Issues of Older Women: A Comprehensive Review for Health Care Professionals* (ed: Victor J. Malatesta) The Haworth Press, Inc., 2007, pp. 31-48. Single or multiple copies of this article are available for a fee from The Haworth Document Delivery Service [1-800-HAWORTH, 9:00 a.m. - 5:00 p.m. (EST). E-mail address: docdelivery@haworthpress.com].

31

tective factor against Coronary Heart Disease and osteoporosis. However, with heavier drinking, these benefits are either reversed or eclipsed. In addition, any alcohol consumption increases the risk for breast cancer in older women. The possible beneficial effects of alcohol must be weighed with the fact that the research does not typically establish causality, that low-risk drinking equates to one standard drink per day, that there is a risk of progression towards alcohol dependence, and that there are alternate methods to gain the same benefits without the associated risks. Older women also experience unique barriers to detection of and treatment for alcohol problems. Current treatment options specifically for older women are limited, though researchers are beginning to address differential treatment response of older women, as well as development of elder women-specific treatment approaches. Treatment options include self-help/mutual peer support, which provides ancillary advantages, brief interventions in primary care settings, which have been demonstrated to be effective in reducing drinking levels, and cognitive behavioral techniques, which have been demonstrated to be useful; but more studies and larger samples are needed. Elder-specific treatments need to be appropriate in terms of content, to address the challenges associated with life stage, such as the loss of the parental role and widowhood, and in terms of process, such as delivery in a respectful therapeutic style and at a slower pace. Future directions in research should address the lack of assessment instruments, the risks of simultaneous use of alcohol and prescription medications, and the under-representation of older women in randomized trials of alcohol treatments.

doi:10.1300/J074v19n01_03 *[Article copies available for a fee from The Haworth Document Delivery Service: 1-800-HAWORTH. E-mail address: <docdelivery@haworthpress.com> Website: <http://www.HaworthPress.com>*

KEYWORDS. Alcohol abuse, alcoholism, aging, women, health

Prevalence of drinking problems declines with age (Sanjuan & Langenbucher, 1999). However, due to less disparity in drinking between men and women at younger ages (Wilsnack & Wilsnack, 1994) as well as other emerging cohort-related factors influencing women's alcohol consumption, the prevalence and impact of older female drinkers is expected to increase as the wave of baby boomers reaches older ages and as current younger generations move toward older adulthood

(Gfroerer, Penne, Pemberton, & Folsom, 2003). Due to differences in metabolism of alcohol compared to men, women of all ages are at higher risk for negative physical, medical, social, and psychological consequences associated with at-risk and higher levels of alcohol consumption. As women age, these risks are intensified; in addition, life span events that typically occur in middle and late adulthood present unique challenges to women in terms of drinking antecedents. Older women also experience unique barriers to detection of and treatment for alcohol problems. Current treatment options specifically for older women are limited, though researchers are beginning to address differential treatment response of older women, as well as development of elder women-specific treatment approaches. This paper provides a description of drinking prevalence, etiology (risk factors), consequences, and treatment challenges for women as they progress through middle and older age.

DEFINITIONS AND PREVALENCE OF ALCOHOL USE DISORDERS AMONG OLDER WOMEN

Among alcohol dependent participants born between 1941 and 1960, those born after 1951 had higher rates of alcohol dependence, with an earlier onset and a longer duration of alcohol-related problems (Holdcraft & Iacono, 2002). The prevalence of alcohol dependence was 21% greater for men from the later cohort than men from the earlier cohort. For women, this difference was 117% greater. According to the latest National Survey on Drug Use and Health by the Substance Abuse and Mental Health Services Administration (SAMHSA, 2004), adult men were almost twice as likely to have a substance-related disorder as women, but among the 12-17 age group the rates were similar for both genders. Thus, as the younger cohort ages, we are likely to see alcohol use problems among more and more females in later life.

Among older women, approximately 75% are abstinent from alcohol (Blow & Barry, 2002). Alcohol use ranges from low-risk to formal diagnoses of alcohol dependence. In a sample of 8578 men and women (n = 3676) ages 55 to 97 (mean age was 68.8) screened in primary care settings (Blow et al., 2000a), 32.94% of men and 29.12% of women were low-risk drinkers. Low-risk drinking as defined by the National Institute on Alcohol Abuse and Alcoholism (NIAAA) is under a limit of one standard drink per day (i.e., 12 ounce domestic beer, 5 ounces of wine, or 1.5 ounces 80 proof liquor), or seven drinks per week, for men and women age 65 and older (U.S. Department of Health and Human Services, 2005). Low-risk use of alcohol is considered non-problematic if not while driving, and not in conjunction with medications that interact negatively with alcohol.

In the Blow et al. (2000a) sample, 10.57% of men and 3.40% of women age 55 and older engaged in at-risk drinking. At-risk drinking was defined here as nine or more drinks per week for women and 12 or more for men, higher than the current NIAAA guidelines of seven drinks per week (1 per day) for men and women over the age of 65. Adams, Barry, and Fleming (1996) found that 12% of women over age 60 in a primary care setting drank more than seven drinks a week.

"Problem drinking" (otherwise known as Hazardous Drinking) is that which has already caused negative consequences for health, family relations, or psychological well-being (Blow & Barry, 2002) but at levels that do not reach formal criteria for an alcohol use disorder.

In the United States, Alcohol Abuse as specified in the Diagnostic and Statistical Manual of Mental Disorders–Fourth Edition (DSM-IV, American Psychiatric Association [APA], 2000) is diagnosed if the person's alcohol use results in or is characterized by at least one of the following recurrently in a 12-month period: (1) failure to fulfill major role obligations at work, school, or home; (2) drinking in situations where use is physically hazardous (e.g., driving while intoxicated); (3) legal problems, or (4) continued use despite alcohol-related interpersonal or social problems. An Alcohol Dependence diagnosis is given based on meeting at least three of seven criteria over a 12-month period involving (1) physical tolerance; (2) physical withdrawal symptoms; (3) loss of control over quantity of or time spent drinking; (4) unsuccessful attempts to cut down, or persistent worry about cutting down; (5) excessive time spent obtaining, using, or recovering from alcohol (10 hours per week is our guideline); (6) substitution of alcohol use for other important social, occupational, or recreational activities; or (7) continued drinking despite knowledge of a recurring alcohol-related physical or psychological problem. Alcohol Dependence with physiological dependence means that the three criteria endorsed include either tolerance or withdrawal.

Data from the National Epidemiologic Survey on Alcohol and Related Conditions (Grant et al., 2004) put the prevalence of alcohol abuse or dependence for women in the past 12 months at .51% for women age 65 and older, 2.85% for women age 45-64, and 5.92% for women age 30-44. For men, the percentages for the same age groups, respectively, are 2.75, 8.17, and 13.67. These rates for women in 2001/02 were approximately double those in 1991 for two age groups, 44-64 and 65 or older, indicating that alcohol use disorders are increasing among more recent cohorts of older women.

Of concern particularly for older women is the oft-prescribed use of sedative drugs such as benzodiazepines as well as barbiturates and anti-depressants (Sanjuan & Langenbucher, 1999), which can interact with alcohol in problematic ways, creating cross-addiction and augmentation of the effects of alcohol in the case of sedatives and barbiturates, and decreased effectiveness of anti-depressants (Blow, 1998). CSAT (1998) reported rates of 11% for women above age 59 who abuse psychoactive drugs.

Blow (2000) has pointed out that rates of any problematic alcohol consumption among older women are likely to be underestimates, given that the measures used are primarily targeted for younger adults and may not be sensitive to alcohol-related sequelae among the elderly. Also, older women may tend to feel more stigmatized by drinking and less likely to disclose rates or habits of alcohol consumption. Estimates are higher (approximately 15% for concurrent alcohol abuse or dependence) among those screened at primary care clinics.

COURSE

Physiologically, women of all ages are more susceptible to the effects of heavy drinking than are men. Because of less body water than men of similar weight, less lean muscle mass, and lower levels of the enzyme that breaks down alcohol in the stomach, women reach higher blood alcohol concentrations than men from the same weight-adjusted levels of alcohol consumption. This results in a "telescoping effect": women develop problems earlier in their drinking careers than men, suffering more severe sequelae from alcohol use and abuse than men, with a shorter latency to developing a host of diseases (Redgrave et al., 2003; Wilsnack & Wilsnack, 1994). For instance, cirrhosis of the liver develops with less alcohol consumption and after a shorter duration of drinking when compared with men (Nolen-Hoeksema, 2004). Evidence for the greater neurotoxicity of alcohol for women than men has been demonstrated by Hommer et al. (2001). As women age, the telescoping effect intensifies, because of decrease of lean tissue, impaired ability to metabolize and clear the alcohol due to compromised hepatic and renal functioning, decreased effectivenss of the blood brain barrier, and increased use of prescription drugs (Sanjuan & Langenbucher, 1999). Thus, even low-risk levels of drinking can be hazardous for older

women. In summary, women are particularly at risk for negative consequences of alcohol, including drug interactions, physical injury from
alcohol-related falls and accidents, cognitive impairment, liver and
heart disease (Blow, 2000).

A distinction has been made between Early and Late Onset Drinking
among older adults. Late adult onset, also known as "reactive" drinking,
has been defined variously as occurring after age 60 (Cowart & Sutherland,
1998), 50 (Schutte, Brennan, & Moos, 1998), and 40 (Gomberg, 1994).
Regardless of the threshold age chosen, late adult onset generally refers to
the start of regular problem drinking. It has been postulated that early adult
onset drinkers present with alcohol-related problems as young adults that
continue into late adulthood, while late adult onset characterizes regular
drinking beginning in response to late life stressors such as retirement, widowhood, isolation, or illness (Blow, 2000; Liberto & Oslin, 1997). While
less than a third of men are late adult onset drinkers with the threshold defined as age 40, over 50% of women were categorized as late adult onset
drinkers (Gomberg, 1995). In terms of predictive validity or clinical utility
of the early versus late adult onset distinction, further research is necessary
as there is no clear consensus in this area.

COMORBIDITY

Alcoholic women are more likely to suffer from anxiety disorders
and depression than alcoholic men, and women in the general population (Petrakis, 2002). There is evidence that substance-using women
have a greater number of comorbid conditions than men (Brennan,
Kagay, Geppert, & Moos, 2000); the National Comorbidity Study
found that alcoholic women reported more comorbid disorders (72.4%)
than men (56.8%) (Grant et al., 2004; Kessler et al., 1997). All of these
gender differences are the same or exacerbated in samples of older
women who drink alcohol problematically. In particular, older women
tend to suffer from depression and abuse of prescribed psychoactive
medication (Gomberg, 1995).

RISK FACTORS FOR DRINKING PROBLEMS
AMONG AGING WOMEN

Women of all ages differ from men in that they are more likely to
drink when alone and to drink in response to a depressed mood. They

also are more likely to drink due to pressure from their partners (Wilsnack & Wilsnack, 1997) and to have partners who drink heavily. Alcoholic women are more likely to report drinking or feeling like drinking when they feel powerless or inadequate than are men (Beckman, 1980). Risk factors particular to the middle age years of 40 to 59 include disruption of marital status, the challenge of menopause, and loss of parental role as children grow up and leave the home. Among women 60 and older, shared drinking activity between retired spouses has been cited as a risk factor for drinking problems, as has widowhood, retirement, and a sparse social network (Gomberg, 1994).

HEALTH AND ALCOHOL CONSUMPTION AMONG AGING WOMEN

There is a growing and important literature on the beneficial and harmful effects of alcohol on women's health, especially aging women who face unique medical challenges in late life due to hormonal changes and the natural aging process even in the absence of alcohol (see Blow et al., 2000). Research has focused primarily on the association of alcohol consumption and cardiovascular disease, cancer, bone disease, neurocognitive deficits, and hepatic problems among older women.

Menopause results in decreased hormone levels, particularly estrogen, which is associated with an increased risk of developing diseases such as Coronary Heart Disease (CHD) and osteoporosis (Register et al., 2002; Tivis & Gavaler, 1994). Some research suggests that low levels of alcohol consumption interact with hormones and impact the risk of developing these postmenopausal diseases and their progression by increasing estrogen levels (Gavaler et al., 1991). Estrogen levels are increased by the conversion of androgens to estrogen through a process called aromotization. Alcohol consumption not only increases aromotization, but it is also thought to decrease the metabolism of estradiol (an estrogen) allowing for more to remain in the bloodstream (Register et al., 2002). A study of 244 postmenopausal women showed that the majority of moderate ("low risk," no more than 1 standard drink per day) drinkers had higher levels of estradiol in comparison to abstainers. The authors concluded that low-risk alcohol consumption is associated with increased estrogen levels in postmenopausal women, which serve as a protective factor against disease associated with menopause. This study also demonstrated that drinking increasing amounts of alcohol does not become increasingly protective (Tivis & Gavaler, 1994).

Coronary heart disease (CHD) is a leading cause of death among both men and women. In general, women are at high risk for CHD only after menopause, due to decreased estrogen levels. Several studies suggest that moderate (1-2 standard drinks per day) alcohol consumption is associated in postmenopausal women with decreased rates of CHD (see Register et al., 2002). For example, Fuchs et al. (1995) compared light (defined as less than 1 drink per day), moderate (up to 2 drinks per day), heavy (more than 2 drinks per day), and non-drinkers and found that overall rates of mortality and mortality due to CHD were less for women who engaged in light to moderate drinking, particularly for those women who had at least one cardiovascular risk factor, whereas rates of CHD for women who engaged in heavy drinking were greater. Furthermore, Davies et al. (2002) found that moderate (defined as 1 drink per day) alcohol consumption by postmenopausal women lowers the risk of CHD by improving cholesterol levels (both HDL and LDL levels), decreasing insulin levels, and increasing insulin sensitivity.

Osteoporosis is a common disease affecting postmenopausal women. It has been implicated in increased susceptibility to fractures, increased rates of disability, increased rates of depression, decreased productivity, and decreased quality of life (Emanuele et al., 2002). By age 35 women achieve peak bone mass that then slowly declines at a rate of approximately 0.5% to 1% annually. At the onset of menopause, bone mass begins to rapidly decline at a rate of approximately 3% to 7% annually (Bonnick, 1994). Lifestyle choices, particularly during adolescence and young adulthood, including regular heavy alcohol consumption, tobacco use, poor nutrition and limited exercise, minimize peak bone mass and bone structure achieved by an individual, and thus heighten the risk for osteoporosis in late adulthood (Sampson, 2002).

Estrogen contributes to the regulation of bone resorption (breakdown) and formation, which helps to maintain bone mass (Emanuele et al., 2002). Feskanich et al. (1999) showed that drinking at "moderate levels" (defined here as 1-2 drinks per day) in postmenopausal women may be associated with greater bone mineral density, and consequent decreased fracture risk in comparison to non-drinkers and heavy drinkers. The authors hypothesize that the health benefits of moderate alcohol consumption may be attributed to increased endogenous estrogens or greater secretion of calcitonin. On the other hand, individuals who drink at heavier levels are at an increased risk for fractures because their bone health is compromised. Their bones tend to be weak and lack density. One explanation is that severe alcoholics tend to be malnourished resulting in vitamin D deficiencies. And, excessive alcohol consumption also results in impairment of balance and consequently fractures due to falling while intoxicated. It appears that other health risks associated with drinking outweigh the possible osteoporitic benefits of low-level drinking.

Although there may be health benefits to low-risk alcohol consumption that increases estrogen levels in postmenopausal women, it is clear that alcohol consumption has detrimental effects (Moos et al., 2004). For example, research has shown that the risk of breast cancer increases with each drink an individual consumes (see Register et al., 2002), though the mechanism is not well understood. Even half a drink per day is associated with increased risk of developing breast cancer. It has been hypothesized that hormone replacement therapy (HRT) intensifies the effect of alcohol. As mentioned above, alcohol increases the amount of estrogen in the system by blocking the breakdown of estradiol; thus, when in combination, use of alcohol and HRT may have a synergistic effect, resulting in high levels of estrogen remaining in the blood for an extended period of time. HRT has been linked with risk of breast cancer. One study found that women who used HRT and drank half a drink or more per day had an increased risk of breast cancer. There was no difference in breast cancer rates between abstainers and moderate drinkers who did not use HRT (Gapstur et al., 1992).

Research on the effects of alcohol consumption on neurocognitive functioning has been mixed (see Sohrabji, 2002). Women who engage in heavy drinking are more susceptible to neurocognitive degeneration as evidenced by brain imaging that shows smaller corpus callosums and larger intracranial spaces (Hommer et al., 2001). Heavy drinking (defined here as more than 3 drinks per day) increases the risk of dementia and memory deficits (Sohrabji, 2002). The role of estrogen in neurocognitive functioning is also questionable. Studies have shown it has a preventative but not a therapeutic effect.

The risk of liver disease may be greater for women who consume as little as two drinks per day (see Kovacs & Messingham, 2002). One explanation is that women metabolize less alcohol in the stomach, which causes an increased blood alcohol level and intensified burden on the liver to process the alcohol thus resulting in greater risk of liver disease. Also, the interaction of hormones and alcohol may increase the risk of developing liver disease in postmenopausal heavy drinkers (Tivis & Gavaler, 1994).

In summary, the effect of alcohol consumption on women's health is debated among researchers. Unfortunately, the "health benefits" of alcohol have been highlighted in the popular press. Some research suggests that alcohol consumption is beneficial to bone and cardiovascular health while other studies point to an association with health risks such as breast cancer, liver disease, and neurocognitive impairment. Overall, it seems that "moderate," also termed "low-risk" alcohol consumption of no more than one standard drink per day for women (U.S. Department of Health and Human Services, 2005) may be associated with some health benefits, while more intense drinking quantity or frequency undoubtedly heightens risk for adverse medical consequences.

Three caveats are important to mention. First, some researchers have erroneously implicated a causal connection of alcohol to positive health effects based on a statistical association of healthier medical status of low-risk drinkers in contrast to abstainers, without taking account of a possible third influential variable (such as degree of mobility, activity, or sociability, for instance) that might account for the relationships between ill health and abstainers or between better health and low-risk drinkers. Thus, alcohol should not be considered "beneficial" or "protective" unless there is a specific causal mechanism articulated and empirically supported to exist. Second, different researchers tend to define "moderate" in various idiosyncratic ways, which has dangerous implications for conclusions the public may draw about how much is safe to drink. The general public is not aware that "low-risk" drinking equals no more than one drink per day, which equals the fairly limited amount of five ounces of wine, one 12-ounce domestic beer, or 1.5 ounces of 80 proof liquor. Thus, people may think they are simply following health guidelines for low-risk levels but actually consuming at-risk, hazardous or problematic levels of alcohol. Any drinking above the low-risk level has health risks and negative consequences for the cardiovascular, skeletal, and reproductive systems, for women of all ages, but is especially deleterious for older women. Third, even if women understand that one standard drink per day is not unhealthy, due to the addictive nature of the substance, which results in tolerance, the quantity and frequency of alcohol consumption might rapidly increase to hazardous or harmful levels over time. Once alcohol dependence has developed, it is difficult to detect and treat, such that a whole new set of medical and psychosocial problems develop, which far outweigh the possible health benefits of one standard drink per day that started the progression towards dependence.

Thus, a recommendation of alcohol consumption as a healthy option for older women should be done only with extreme caution, and limits of quantity should be made clear (i.e., "no more than five ounces of wine per day and you should use a measuring cup" rather than "drink a glass a day." The amount and type of alcohol consumed, as well as personal and family history of alcohol problems, should be taken into consideration when weighing the costs and benefits of advising or heeding advice to drink regularly as a health enhancement. For instance, Barry et al. (2001) recommend that professionals not advocate therapeutic alcohol use for patients who never drank before, or for those who have a history of problematic drinking. Other alternatives to similar therapeutic effects to the same organ systems without the possible risks of alcohol use are regular aerobic and weight-bearing exercise, healthy balanced diet, and positive attitudes. De-alcoholized red wine, red wine, and grape juice most of all have been shown to inhibit the buildup of plaque in arteries in hamsters (Vinson, Teufel, & Wu, 2001).

IDENTIFICATION AND TREATMENT OF ALCOHOL USE PROBLEMS IN OLDER WOMEN

Barriers to Detection and Treatment

Women are more likely to approach general health-care facilities for their problem drinking than alcohol specific treatment programs, and to appear with more severe symptoms than men (Thom, 1986; Weisner & Schmidt, 1992). They also are more likely than men to present depression and anxiety as their main problem (Bijl & Ravelli, 2000; Proudfoot & Teesson, 2002; Wu, Kouzis, & Leaf, 1999). In a review of general barriers to help-seeking, Schober and Annis (1996) found that women entering treatment are more likely than men to experience personal shame and embarrassment. They are less likely to have insurance coverage (Estes, 1995), and drink primarily at home alone so are not likely to be identified as a problem drinker by family and friends who then might encourage them to seek treatment. On the other hand, older women are more likely than men to seek medical care (Fleming & Barry, 1992), so this opens an opportunity for health-care professionals to screen for alcohol use problems (Blow, 2000). Health-care providers in general do not assume that older women drink alcohol problematically and do not screen for this (Blow & Barry, 2002).

Recommended Assessment Tools

Blow (1998, 2000) recommends routine screening for alcohol and prescription drug abuse in primary health-care settings for older women (over 60), and the use of elder-specific measures to screen for alcohol use problems, such as the Michigan Alcoholism Screening Test–Geriatric Version (MAST-G; Blow et al., 1992), or the Alcohol Use Disorders Identification Test (AUDIT, Babor & Grant, 1992) which has been validated on older samples (Barry, Oslin, & Blow, 2001). Screening should be done annually, as well as before prescribing any new medications that may interact with alcohol, and also as needed after life-changing or stressful events such as death of a spouse. Screening questions should cover alcohol consumption (quantity and frequency), physical and social consequences, medication use and interaction with alcohol, and depression (Adams, Barry, & Fleming, 1996; Blow & Barry, 2002).

Barry et al. (2001) lists the following as possibly indicative of drinking problems among older women: anxiety, tolerance to alcohol or medication, depression or mood swings, memory problems, disorientation, difficulty making decisions, poor hygiene, falls, bruises or burns, family problems, seizures of an unknown origin, financial problems, sleep difficulty, headaches, social isolation, incontinence, and poor nutrition. It is clear from this list that differential diagnosis of alcohol use problems can be difficult among the elderly, as most if not all of these problems listed can multiply or otherwise be determined. Thus, direct questions that are designed to minimize denial are suggested, and are to be administered as part of a larger battery of health related questions. For instance, instead of asking, "do you drink alcohol?" ask "How many times per week do you drink an alcoholic beverage." If the answer is none, then ask "How many times per month?" It is important to understand that older women are likely to minimize their drinking and related symptoms. Asking not only about frequency of alcohol consumption but also about quantity consumed (in standard drinks) is important to help the clinician understand the extent and possible negative consequences of the patient's alcohol use regardless of her self-report. The clinician can estimate blood alcohol levels based on report of quantity, time spent drinking, and weight of the patient, in order to help determine level of intoxication the woman is attaining and associated risks such as stumbling, memory problems, etc. (Roberts & McCrady, 2003). Blood tests to assess hepatic function (GGTP, AST, ALT, Bilirubin) and presence of other substances in the system can also be used to identify alcohol and other drug problems. Alcohol counselors also need to screen for other health problems and use of estrogen replacement therapy to help determine the risks associated with alcohol use.

Treatment of Alcohol Use Disorders in Older Women

Older women can avail themselves of self-help and treatment options open to all individuals who have an alcohol problem; this includes a range of care from inpatient detoxification and inpatient rehabilitation programs, to outpatient management of detoxification, intensive outpatient programs (9 hours a week) or weekly individual or group psychotherapy. The advantages of self-help/mutual peer support groups are wide availability, no cost, and social interaction that can facilitate alleviation of loneliness and practical problems such as rides to meetings. Currently there are mutual peer support groups that cater specifically to women, such as Alcoholics Anonymous women's groups and Women for Sobriety, but no self-help groups that particularly address concerns of older adults or older women in particular. Formal treatments have historically been developed and tested on male samples, though in the past 10 years there has been increasing focus on development of female-specific treatment approaches. In terms of elder-specific treatment approaches, brief interventions in primary care settings (Barry et al., 2001; Fleming et al., 1999; Blow & Barry, 2002) with older at-risk and hazardous drinkers, have been shown to reduce drinking frequency of both men and women. In addition, cognitive behavioral programs that teach skills to cope with problems of older adulthood such as grief and loneliness, case management approaches, and elder-specific programming to help older alcohol dependent individuals have been found to be useful (Atkinson, 1995; Blow et al., 2000a; Schonfeld et al., 2000), but studies have been few and samples have been small. Additional research is needed to continue to test and develop elder-specific and especially elder female-specific programs. There is some evidence that older women may respond to alcohol treatment better than older men. For instance, Satre et al. (2004) found that of 92 patients (29 women) age 55-77, who engaged in a 12-month outpatient day hospital or less intensive outpatient group and individual treatment program, a higher percentage of females (79.3%) were abstinent from alcohol and drugs at six-month follow up than males (54%). Men also reported more heavy drinking days than the women at follow-up.

Elder-specific treatment programs target both age-related content and treatment venues and modality. For instance, sites such as primary care settings are ideal venues in which to develop elder-specific treatments, especially for women who are more likely to seek medical treatment than are men. In terms of designing elder-specific therapy, Blow et al. (2000a) list issues that older adults tend to face and need to address in therapy, such as loss, isolation, health problems, and grief. Other older adult life span relevant topics such as worries about the future of independent living, menopause, grandparenting, retirement, decreased mobility, depression, fixed income, and life review would also be appropriate for elder-specific therapy for alcohol use disorders. In addition to therapy content, Blow et al. (2000a) describe therapy process variables important for elder-specific programs: respectful rather than confrontational approaches, accommodation for impaired hearing, accommodation of medical needs, bolstering of therapeutic alliance with younger therapists who need to be aware of issues facing older adults, slower pace of treatment, case management, addressing spiritual needs of the patients, and tailoring of treatment to level of cognitive functioning of each patient. It is also recommended that elder female-specific therapy include aspects of the emerging positive psychology approach, such that not only are problems targeted, emotions explored and coping skills taught, but also the importance of developing and maintaining an optimistic and positive attitude toward one's life and one's self is stressed and how to keep busy with interesting and enriching activities as alternatives to drinking.

NEED FOR ADDITIONAL RESEARCH AND RESOURCES FOR FURTHER STUDY

Based on initial promising effects of brief interventions in primary care settings to identify and help patients reduce hazardous and at-risk drinking, Blow and Barry (2002) recommend further research to determine active ingredients, and other sites of treatment such as in-home health care or senior centers. In addition, research on simultaneous use of alcohol and prescription medications is necessary to determine specific risks and treatments, since this is a prominent pattern of use among older women. It is recommended that older women be over-selected to participate in randomized studies of alcohol treatments so that this population in these samples can be adequately represented. More research is needed to assess which treatments, such as elder female-specific programs, would be most effective for older women. In addition, development of age- and gender-specific and appropriate assessment instruments should be a target of research efforts (Blow,

2000). Oslin et al. (2005) reported that older adults did as well as middle aged adults after alcohol treatment but did not make as much use of aftercare; this would also be an important area to target for older women especially who may benefit from longer-term post-treatment affiliation with a therapy program.

In terms of future research on possible health benefits of alcohol use, it would be important to ameliorate some problems with research to date. First, the majority of the studies are not randomized clinical trials but are naturalistic designs. Second, researchers rely on self-report measures of alcohol consumption, which are often inaccurate. Third, control groups often consist of abstainers who are different from drinkers in terms of habits (e.g., tobacco use among drinkers), socioeconomic status, health risks, level of social activity and mobility, and history of medical problems. Further research using carefully matched groups is necessary.

REFERENCES

Adams, W., Barry, K.L., & Fleming, M.F. (1996). Screening for alcohol use in older primary care patients. *Journal of the American Medical Association, 279,* 1964-1967.

American Psychiatric Association (2000). *Diagnostic and statistical manual of mental disorders,* fourth Edition, text revision (DSM-IV-TR). Washington, DC.

Atkinson, R.M. (1995). Treatment programs for aging alcoholics. In T. Beresford & E. Gomberg (Eds.), *Alcohol and aging.* New York: Oxford University Press, 186- 210.

Babor, T., & Grant, M. (1992). *Project on identification and management of alcohol-related problems. Report on Phase II: A randomized clinical trial of brief interventions in primary health care.* Geneva: World Health Organization.

Baer, D.J., Judd, J.T., Clevidence, B.A., Muesing, R.A., Campbell, W.S., Brown, E.D. et al. (2002). *American Journal of Clinical Nutrition, 75*(3), 593-599.

Barry, K.L., Oslin, D.W., & Blow, F.C. (2001). *Alcohol problems in older adults: Prevention and management.* New York: Springer Publishing Company, Inc.

Blow, F.C. (1998). *Substance abuse among older americans (DHHS No. (SMA) 98-3179).* Washington, DC: U.S. Government Printing Office.

Blow, F.C. (2000). Treatment of older women with alcohol problems: Meeting the challenge for a special population. *Alcoholism: Clinical and Experimental Research, 24*(8), 1257-1266.

Blow, F.C., & Barry, K.L. (2002). Use and misuse of alcohol among older women. *Alcohol Research and Health, 26*(4), 308-315.

Blow, F.C., Brower, K.J., Schulenberg, J.E., Demo-Dananberg, L.M., Young, J.P., & Beresford, T.P. (1992). The Michigan Alcoholism Screening Test–Geriatric Version (MAST-G): A new elderly-specific screening instrument. *Alcoholism: Clinical and Experimental Research, 16,* 372.

Blow, F.C., Walton, M.A. Barry, K.L., Coyne, J.C., Mudd, S.A., & Copeland, L.A. (2000). The relationship between alcohol problems and health functioning of older adults in primary care settings. *Journal of the American Geriatric Society, 48*(7), 769-774.

Blow, F.C., Walton, M.A., Chermack, S.T., Mudd, S.A., & Brower, K.J. (2000). Older adult treatment outcome following elder-specific inpatient alcoholism treatment. *Journal of Substance Abuse Treatment, 19*, 67-75.

Bonnick, S.L. (1994). *The osteoporosis handbook.* Dallas: Taylor Publishing.

Brennan, P.L., Kagay, C.R., Geppert, J.J., & Moos, R.H. (2000). Elderly medicare inpatients with substance use disorders: Characteristics and predictors of hospital readmissions over a four-year interval. *Journal of Studies on Alcohol, 61*(6), 891-895.

Center for Substance Abuse Treatment (1998). *Treatment improvement protocol #26: substance abuse among older adults.* F. C. Blow, DHHS No. (SMA)98-3179. Center for Substance Abuse Treatment, Rockville, MD.

Cowart, M.E., & Sutherland, M. (1998). Late life drinking among women. *Geriatric Nursing, 19*(4), 214-219.

Davies, M.J., Baer, D.J., Judd, J.T., Brown, E.D., Campbell, W.S., & Taylor, P.R. (2002). Effects of moderate alcohol intake on fasting insulin and glucose concentrations and insulin sensitivity in postmenopausal women: A randomized controlled trial. *Journal of the American Medical Association, 287*(19), 2559-2562.

Emanuele, M., Wezeman, F., & Emanuele, N. (2002). Alcohol's effects on female reproductive function. *Alcohol and Research World, 26*(4), 274-281.

Estes, C.L. (1995). Mental health services for the elderly: Key policy elements. In M. Gatz (Ed.), *Emerging Issues in Mental Health and Aging.* American Psychological Association, Washington, DC, 301-318.

Feskanich, D., Korrick, S., Greenspan, S., Rosen, H., & Colditz, G. (1999). Moderate alcohol consumption and bone density among postmenopausal women. *Journal of Women's Health, 8*(1), 65-73.

Fleming, M.L., & Barry, K.L. (Eds.) (1992). *Addictive disorders: A practical guide to treatment.* St. Louis, MO: Mosby/Yearbook Medical Publishers.

Fleming, M.L., Manwell, L.B., Barry, K.L., & Adams, W. (1999). Brief physician advice for alcohol problems in older adults: A randomized community-based trial. *Journal of Family Practice, 48*, 378-384.

Fuchs, C.S., Stampfer, M.J., Colditz, G.A., Giovannucci, E.L., Manson, J.E., Kawachi, I. et al. (1995). Alcohol consumption and mortality among women. *The New England Journal of Medicine, 332*(19), 1245-1250.

Gapstur, S.M., Potter, J.D., Sellers, T.A., & Folsom, A.R. (1992). Increased risk of breast cancer with alcohol consumption in postmenopausal women. *American Journal of Epidemiology 136*(10), 1221-1231.

Gfroerer, J., Penne, M., Pemberton, M., & Folsom, R. (2003). Substance abuse treatment need among older adults in 2020: The impact of the aging baby-boom cohort. *Drug and Alcohol Dependence, 69*, 127-135.

Gomberg, E.S.L. (1994). Risk factors for drinking over a woman's life span. *Alcohol Health and Research World, 18*(3), 220-289.

Gomberg, E.S.L. (1995). Older women and alcohol use and abuse. *Recent Developments in Alcohol, 12*, 61-79.

Grant, B.F., Dawson, D.A., Stinson, F.S., Chou, S.P., Dufour, M.C., & Pickering, R.P. (2004). The 12-month prevalence and trends in DSM-IV alcohol abuse and dependence: United States, 1991-1992 and 2001-2002. *Drug and Alcohol Dependence, 74*(3), 223-234.

Grant, B.F., Stinson, F.S., Dawson, D.A., Chou, S.P., Ruan, W.J., & Pickering, R.P. (2004a). Co-occurrence of 12-month alcohol and drug use disorders and personality disorders in the United States: Results from the national epidemiologic survey on alcohol and related conditions. *Arch Gen Psychiatry, 61*(4), 361-368.

Holdcraft, L.C., & Iacono, W.G. (2002). Cohort effects on gender differences in alcohol dependence. *Addiction, 97*(8), 1025-1036.

Hommer, D., Momenan, R., Kaiser, E., & Rawlings, R. (2001). Evidence for gender-related effect of alcoholism on brain volumes. *American Journal of Psychiatry, 158*(2), 198-204.

Kessler, R.C., Crum, R.M., Warner, L.A., Nelson, C.B., Schulenberg, J., & Anthony, J.C. (1997). Lifetime co-occurrence of DSM-III-R alcohol abuse and dependence with other psychiatric disorders in the national comorbidity survey. *Arch Gen Psychiatry, 54*(4), 313-321.

Kovacs, E.J., & Messingham, K. (2002). Influence of alcohol and gender on immune response. *Alcohol and Research World, 26*(4), 257-263.

Liberto, J.G., & Oslin, D.W. (1995). Early versus late onset of alcoholism in the elderly. *International Journal of the Addictions, 30*(13-14), 1799-1818.

Liberto, J.G., & Oslin, D.W. (1997), Early versus late onset of alcoholism in the elderly. In A.M. Gurnack (Ed.), *Older adults' misuse of alcohol, medicines, and other drugs: Research and practice issues.* New York: Spring Publishing Co., 94-112.

Liberto, J.G., Oslin, D.W., & Ruskin, P.E. (1992). Alcoholism in older persons: A review of the literature. *Hospital Community Psychiatry, 43*, 975-984.

Moos, R.H., Brennan, P.L., Schutte, K.K., & Moos, B.S. (2004). High risk alcohol consumption and late-life alcohol use problems. *American Journal of Public Health, 94* (11), 1985-1991.

Nolen-Hoeksema, S. (2004). Gender differences in risk factors and consequences for alcohol use and problems. *Clinical Psychology Review, 24*(8), 981-1010.

Oslin, D.W., Slaymaker, V.J., Blow, F.C., Owen, P.L., & Colleran, C. (2005). Treatment outcomes for alcohol dependence among middle-aged and older adults. *Addictive Behaviors, 30*, 1431-1436.

Petrakis, I.L.G., Gerardo, Rosenheck, Robert, & Krystal, John H. (2002). Comorbidity of alcoholism and psychiatric disorders: An overview. *Alcohol Research and Health, 26*(2), 81-89.

Proudfoot, H., & Teesson, M. (2002). Who seeks treatment for alcohol dependence? *Social Psychiatry & Psychiatric Epidemiology, 37*(10), 451-456.

Redgrave, G.W., Swartz, K.L., & Romanoski, A.J. (2003). Alcohol misuse by women. *International Review of Psychiatry, 15*(3), 256-268.

Register, T.C., Cline, M., & Shively, C.A. (2002). Health issues in postmenopausal women who drink. *Alcohol and Research World, 26*(4), 299-307.

Roberts, L.J. & McCrady, B.S. (2003). *Alcohol problems in intimate relationships: Identification and intervention. A guide for marriage and family therapists.* NIH

Publication No. 03-5284. Bethesda, MD: National Institute on Alcohol Abuse and Alcoholism.

Sampson, W.S. (2002). Alcohol and other factors affecting osteoporosis risk in women. *Alcohol and Research World, 26*(4), 292-298.

Sanjuan, P.M., & Langenbucher, J.W. (1999). Age-limited populations: Youth, adolescents, and older adults. In B.S. McCrady & E.E. Epstein (Eds.), *Addictions: A comprehensive guidebook.* New York: Oxford University Press, 477-498.

Satre, D.D., Mertens, J.R., & Weisner, C. (2004). Gender differences in treatment outcomes for alcohol dependence among older adults. *Journal of Studies on Alcohol, 65,* 5, 638-642.

Schober, R., & Annis, H.M. (1996). Barriers to help-seeking for change in drinking: A gender-focused review of the literature. *Addictive Behaviors, 21,* 81-92.

Schonfeld, I., Dupree, I.W., Dickson-Fuhrmann, E. et al. (2000). Cognitive-behavioral treatment of older veterans with substance use problems. *Journal of Geriatric Psychiatry and Neurology, 13*(3), 124-129.

Schutte, K., Brennan, P., & Moos, R. (1998). Predicting the development of late-life late-onset drinking problems: A 7-year prospective study. *Alcoholism: Clinical and Experimental Research, 22,* 1349-1358.

Sohrabji, F. (2002). Neurodegeneration in women. *Alcohol and Research World, 26*(4), 3116-318.

Substance Abuse and Mental Health Services Administration, Office of Applied Studies (2004). *National survey of substance abuse treatment services (N-SSATS): 2003. Data on substance abuse treatment facilities.* DASIS Series: S-24, DHHS Publication No. (SMA) 04-3966. Rockville, MD.

Thom, B. (1986). Sex differences in help-seeking for alcohol problems-1. The barriers to help-seeking. *British Journal of Addiction, 81,* 777-788.

Tivis, L.J., & Gavaler, J.S. (1994). Alcohol, hormones, and health in postmenopausal women. *Alcohol and Research World, 18*(3), 185-189.

U.S. Department of Health and Human Services, National Institutes of Health (2005). *Alcohol: A woman's health issue.* NIH Publication number 03-4956.

Vinson, J.A., Teufel, K., & Wu, N. (2001). Red wine, dealcoholized red wine, and especially grape juice, inhibit atherosclerosis in a hamster model. *Atherosclerosis, 156*(1), 67-72.

Weisner, C., & Schmidt, L. (1992). Gender disparities in treatment for alcohol problems. *JAMA, 268*(14), 1872-1876.

Wilsnack, R.W., & Wilsnack, S.C. (Eds.) (1997). *Gender and alcohol: Individual and social perspectives.* Piscataway, NJ: Rutgers Center of Alcohol Studies.

Wilsnack, S.C., & Wilsnack, R.W. (1994). How women drink: Epidemiology of women's drinking and problem drinking. *Alcohol Health and Research World, 18*(3), 173-181.

Wu, L.-T., Kouzis, A.C., & Leaf, P.J. (1999). Influence of comorbid alcohol and psychiatric disorders on utilization of mental health services in the national comorbidity survey. *American Journal of Psychiatry, 156*(8), 1230-1236.

doi:10.1300/J074v19n01_03

Women, Aging, and Schizophrenia

Faith B. Dickerson, PhD, MPH

SUMMARY. Schizophrenia is a psychiatric disorder of unknown etiology that typically has an onset in early adulthood and persists for the remainder of the life span. For most affected individuals, the illness is recurrent with psychotic symptoms that tend to be episodic in nature. The illness has pervasive and disruptive effects on many life domains; for example, women with schizophrenia are less likely to marry, bear children, and raise their own children than are women in the general population. The age of onset of schizophrenia is later on average in women than men, and women are overrepresented among those who develop the illness after the age of 45. Among younger patients with schizophrenia, women tend to have less severe symptoms than men and better outcomes; however, there are fewer gender differences among older patients with schizophrenia. Older women with schizophrenia are vulnerable to problems of both schizophrenia and aging. Schizophrenia symptoms typically continue in later years and include ongoing psychotic symptoms. Problems of aging such as cognitive decline and chronic medical conditions may be exacerbated by schizophrenia and the disorder is associated with premature mortality. Older women with schizophrenia are at risk for neglect of psychiatric and

Address correspondence to: Faith B. Dickerson, Sheppard Pratt, 6501 North Charles Street, Baltimore, MD 21201 (E-mail: fdickerson@sheppardpratt.org).

[Haworth co-indexing entry note]: "Women, Aging, and Schizophrenia." Dickerson, Faith B. Co-published simultaneously in *Journal of Women & Aging* (The Haworth Press, Inc.) Vol. 19, No. 1/2, 2007, pp. 49-61; and: *Mental Health Issues of Older Women: A Comprehensive Review for Health Care Professionals* (ed: Victor J. Malatesta) The Haworth Press, Inc., 2007, pp. 49-61. Single or multiple copies of this article are available for a fee from The Haworth Document Delivery Service [1-800-HAWORTH, 9:00 a.m. - 5:00 p.m. (EST). E-mail address: docdelivery@haworthpress.com].

other health needs that are further compounded by limited social support and low socioeconomic status. More research and clinical attention is needed for the problems of older women with schizophrenia.

doi:10.1300/J074v19n01_04 *[Article copies available for a fee from The Haworth Document Delivery Service: 1-800-HAWORTH. E-mail address: <docdelivery@haworthpress.com> Website: <http://www.HaworthPress.com> © 2007 by The Haworth Press, Inc. All rights reserved.]*

KEYWORDS. Schizophrenia, aging, women, psychosis, serious mental illness

INTRODUCTION

Schizophrenia is a serious psychiatric disorder that in older women is typically a continuation of an illness first experienced during the younger adult years. Studies have examined gender differences in schizophrenia (e.g., Seeman, 2004) and there is a growing interest in middle aged and older adults with the disorder (e.g., Jeste et al., 2003). However, there has been only limited attention to the specific needs and problems of older women with schizophrenia. The following sections present an overview of schizophrenia diagnosis, prevalence, course, and treatment with special reference to women and the aging process.

DESCRIPTION AND DIAGNOSIS

Schizophrenia is a psychiatric disorder that typically has an onset in early adulthood and persists for the remainder of the life span. With pervasive effects on a person's life and over a time period of decades, schizophrenia is arguably the most severe psychiatric disorder. Schizophrenia has diverse manifestations; the diagnosis may be made on the basis of a number of signs and symptoms, and no single clinical feature is pathognomonic (Carpenter & Buchanan, 1994). In general, the diagnosis requires two or more characteristic psychotic symptoms that must be present for a significant portion of a one-month period. In addition to meeting symptom criteria, the diagnosis also requires that a person have had the characteristic symptoms or milder manifestations continuously for at least six months. The person must also have had a decline in occupational or social functioning. Schizophrenia is a diagnosis of exclusion; that is, a medical condition or a primary mood disorder which may account for the symptoms must be ruled out (APA, 1994).

Schizophrenia symptoms may be divided into three major categories. The first category consists of "positive" symptoms which refer to a loss of reality as manifest in the person having false beliefs, known as delusions, or having perceptual or sensory experiences not shared by others, known as hallucinations. Bizarre behaviors also fall in this category. Second are the so-called "negative" symptoms which refer to the absence of some basic, expected emotions or behaviors. Low social drive, poor motivation, and emotional flattening fall in this category. In the overall course of the disorder, these symptoms are often the most debilitating. The third major category of symptoms is that of disorganization and refers to speech which is tangential or incoherent, and impaired attention. It is important to emphasize that not all persons with schizophrenia have all of the symptoms associated with the disorder and that the persons with the diagnosis may present with various combinations of the symptoms described above.

The diagnostic manual defines subtypes of schizophrenia including paranoid and disorganized types but the subtypes do not represent robust distinctions that determine clinical treatment. Schizoaffective disorder is a related disorder that is frequently grouped with schizophrenia. Schizoaffective disorder refers to a person who meets the diagnostic criteria for schizophrenia and also meets criteria for a major mood disorder; in addition, symptoms of delusions or hallucinations must be present for at least two weeks in the absence of prominent mood symptoms (APA, 1994).

Schizophrenia is associated with other psychiatric and clinical problems which are not part of the diagnostic criteria for schizophrenia but which are more prevalent in individuals with schizophrenia than in the general population. These frequent co-occurring problems include depression, anxiety, and also alcohol and drug abuse. Cognitive impairment is increasingly recognized as a problem in schizophrenia including problems in learning, memory, and abstract reasoning. Co-occurring medical illnesses such as type 2 diabetes, respiratory ailments, and cardiovascular problems are also found more often in schizophrenia and there is a higher risk for premature mortality from both natural and unnatural causes (Brown, 1997; Sokal et al., 2004).

Schizophrenia signs and symptoms in older women are similar to those found in younger patients and in male patients; the effects of age and gender on the illness will be discussed in the following sections. The clinical problems experienced by older women with schizophrenia are summarized in Table 1.

TABLE 1. Symptoms and Problems Experienced by Older Women with Schizophrenia[1]

Schizophrenia illness symptoms
Positive symptoms
Negative symptoms[2]
Disorganization
Other psychiatric problems
Depression[3]
Anxiety[3]
Trauma related problems[3]
Cognitive impairment[4]
Alcohol and drug abuse[2]
Medical comorbidity and mortality
Diabetes[4]
Cardiovascular illness[4]
Suicide[2]
Death by accident[2]
Poor Health Behaviors
Smoking
Obesity
Social problems
Unemployment[2]
Poverty and low socioeconomic status
Limited social network and support

[1] All of these symptoms and problems are more prevalent in older women with schizophrenia than in the general population though are not necessarily present in all older women with schizophrenia
[2] Less likely in women than men with schizophrenia
[3] More likely in women than men with schizophrenia
[4] More likely in older than younger persons with schizophrenia

PREVALENCE

The lifetime risk of schizophrenia is approximately 0.7% or 7 per 1000 people (Kessler et al., 1994) and the prevalence is about the same in men and women. Approximately 67% of individuals who go on to develop schizophrenia have done so by age 40; 13% have their onset during their 40s; 7% during their 50s and 3% after age 60 (Harris & Jeste, 1988). However, the average age of onset is several years older in women then in men and the majority of late onset cases, after the age of 45, are women (Lindamer et al., 1999). Therefore, the ratio of men to women in new onset cases varies considerably by age. For example, for those individuals diagnosed in the 15-25 age range, there are 12 men to 10 women; in the 25-35 age range, the ratio of men to women is about even, but after age 35, the preponderance of new cases consists of women though the absolute number of such cases is small (Seeman, 2004).

The reasons for the later onset of schizophrenia in women than in men, and for the preponderance of women among late onset cases, are unknown. One explanation involves the fact that males are more physically vulnerable to environmental insults at birth and also are more likely to sustain head trauma. Another explanation involves the role of estrogen, a female hormone, which may serve a protective role and delay illness onset; also, the decline of estrogen during menopause may lead to some new cases when the protective hormonal effect is lost (Harris & Jeste, 1988). Although late onset cases differ from other cases in the timing of the illness presentation, the signs and symptoms of schizophrenia in late onset cases do not differ significantly from earlier onset cases. Nor is there any overall difference between men and women who develop the illness after the age of 40 (Lehmann, 2003; Howard et al., 2000).

COURSE

There is wide variability in the outcome of schizophrenia, but for most individuals the illness is recurrent with symptoms that tend to be episodic in nature. A portion of patients with schizophrenia, about 25%, evidence good functioning and recovery after the first episode. As many as 25-40% of individuals, however, experience persistent psychotic symptoms despite treatment with antipsychotic medication; for as many as 5-15%, these continuous symptoms are severe (Hegarty et al., 1994; Torrey, 2001). There are a number of factors that contribute to the illness course including the individual's pre-morbid social functioning, the confounding effects of substance abuse, and the degree of adherence to prescribed medication (Mueser & McGurk, 2004). However, these factors do not enable any accurate prediction of outcome for individual cases.

Although the course of schizophrenia is generally similar in men and in women, there are some differences which are of interest. As a group, women with schizophrenia tend to have better premorbid adjustment, perhaps related to their average later age of onset. Accordingly, outcomes are somewhat more benign for affected women in terms of less severe symptoms, lower rates of suicide and accidental death, and better occupational and interpersonal functioning (Bardenstein & McGlashan, 1990; Seeman, 2004). However, for women as well as men there is a lot of inter-individual variability.

Among younger patients with schizophrenia, women tend to have less severe symptoms than men and they also have fewer and shorter hospitalizations. However, there are fewer gender differences among older patients with schizophrenia, perhaps because more of the severely ill men than women have already died (Seeman, 2004; Sajatovic et al., 2002). For both older women and older men with schizophrenia, positive symptoms may diminish with advancing age. One study carried out in Vermont in the 1980s indicated that many persons with schizophrenia evidenced a recovery from the illness during their older years when followed up 20-25 years after hospitalization (Harding et al., 1987). Other research evidence suggests that age does not markedly alter the individual's course of the illness, at least among patients who stay in a treatment system. In one study of nearly 300 older patients aged 40-85 living in community settings, 60% of the patients remained stable, 20% had a worsening of symptoms with age, and 20% had a symptom remission (Jeste et al., 2003).

As patients with schizophrenia age, they are more vulnerable to the spectrum of medical problems including cardiovascular, respiratory, neurological diseases and cancer, as are older persons without schizophrenia (Lehmann, 2003). For patients in outpatient settings, the mild cognitive impairment found at the time of schizophrenia onset appears to remain stable throughout the illness course without marked change as patients age. A different pattern is found among institutionalized patients with schizophrenia, who by definition are a more severely ill group. Unlike patients with schizophrenia living in the community, these patients show a strikingly high prevalence of cognitive impairment and dementia (Harvey et al., 1999).

The personal and reproductive histories of women with schizophrenia are often related to the illness either directly or indirectly. As a group, women with schizophrenia are less likely to marry than women in the general population. They are more prone to experience sexual assault and victimization in general (Miller, 1997; Miller & Finnerty, 1996). They also have fewer pregnancies and live births (Miller & Finnerty, 1996; Dickerson et al., 2004). In addition to reduced childbearing, women with schizophrenia who do have children are more likely to have their children reared by persons other than themselves (Miller & Finnerty, 1996). Mothers with schizophrenia may have difficulty raising their children because of the disruptive effects of their illness symptoms and also the poverty that often is found among persons with the illness. Despite not infrequent custody loss, many mothers with schizophrenia consider motherhood a central role in their lives (Miller, 1997).

ETIOLOGY

The definitive causes of schizophrenia are unknown; a full discussion of this complex topic is beyond the scope of this article. Genetic factors play some role in the disorder in that there is a higher prevalence of schizophrenia in the family members of individuals with schizophrenia than in the population at large. Among first degree relatives (that is, parent, child, sibling) the rate of schizophrenia is 10%, or about 10-fold the risk in the general population. Among offspring of parents who both have schizophrenia, the risk of schizophrenia is 40%. For monozygotic twins, one of whom has schizophrenia, the pairwise concordance of schizophrenia is about 30% (Torrey, 1992). The relatively high discordance between monozygotic twins indicates that while schizophrenia has a significant genetic component, other, environmental, factors must also be at work. If schizophrenia were a completely genetic disease, one would expect to see a nearly 100% concordance between monozygotic twins. Intensive scientific efforts have been directed at defining the genes involved in schizophrenia transmission. Different chromosomal abnormalities have been reported by different researchers and but as yet no highly reliable candidate schizophrenia gene has emerged (Sawa & Snyder, 2002).

In addition to genetics, several environmental factors potentially relevant to schizophrenia etiology have been identified (Mueser & McGurk, 2004). Prenatal and/or perinatal events may play some role in the development of schizophrenia as there is a higher than expected rate of schizophrenia in individuals who have had obstetrical complications with hypoxia at birth. Population migration is also associated with schizophrenia in that some ethnic groups with members who have moved from one country to another country show an unusually high rate of schizophrenia; this phenomenon is found among second generation

Afro-Caribbeans in the United Kingdom, and Dutch Antilleans and Surinamese in Holland. At a population level, other variables that have been associated with schizophrenia are winter births; birthplace in an urban area; and lower social class. While these factors show significant associations at a group or population level, they are not useful in defining the degree of individual risk or determining with any certainty which persons will develop schizophrenia. Another set of environmental factors that has been identified relates to exposure to infectious agents (Yolken & Torrey, 1995; Leweke et al., 2004). There is some data to suggest that an active or inactive viral infection may set the stage for vulnerability to schizophrenia. It is possible that exposure of the affected individual may lead to schizophrenia susceptibility or that the influence may be through maternal infection before or at the time of birth. It is important to note that psychosocial theories of causation of schizophrenia, which were dominant in the mid-twentieth century, have largely been abandoned for lack of evidence.

Just as the causes of schizophrenia have not been delineated, the pathophysiology of the disorder has not yet been identified. While there is overwhelming evidence that the basis of schizophrenia is biological, it is not certain the specific ways in which the central nervous system is abnormal or how such abnormalities then lead to schizophrenia symptoms. One theory is that abnormalities in proteins with key roles in brain development may contribute to the disorder, but the details of this process have not been fully elucidated. Contributing evidence comes from the fact that brain ventricles are relatively enlarged in individuals with schizophrenia; in addition, there are overall reductions in brain volume and in cortical grey matter (Carpenter & Buchanan, 1994). Both of these findings have been observed at the time of schizophrenia onset, so cannot be attributed to illness treatment or course. Abnormalities in blood flow in some brain regions while patients are performing cognitive tasks have also been found (Mueser & McGurk, 2004). While of interest in studying the underpinnings of schizophrenia, these group differences between individuals with schizophrenia and healthy controls are not specific or sensitive enough to be useful in the diagnostic assessment of individual patients.

ASSESSMENT AND TREATMENT RECOMMENDATIONS

The diagnosis of schizophrenia is made by a trained mental health clinician on the basis of the patient's self-report of symptoms, observations of the patient, and reports from collateral sources such as family members. Because of the complexity of the diagnosis and the different inclusion and exclusion criteria, some of which involve duration of symptoms, a diagnosis may be difficult to make based on a cross-sectional assessment. In addition, patients with psychosis may have limited insight about their symptoms and their behavior, so information from patient self-report is not always reliable. It may be necessary to follow the patient for several months after the time that psychotic symptoms first present in order to confirm the diagnosis. As noted earlier, there is no biological or psychological test that is sensitive or specific for schizophrenia. Because the vast majority of patients who go on to develop schizophrenia have done so by age 40, the question of whether the diagnosis is present or not is not likely to be uncertain for older women with schizophrenia.

Antipsychotic medication is the cornerstone of treatment for schizophrenia (Lehman et al., 2004). Other types of medications are also often prescribed such as antidepressants and anticonvulsant mood stabilizers. Antipsychotic medication is not curative but is helpful in reducing schizophrenia symptoms, increasing the likelihood of stability, and reducing the rate of relapse by greater than 50% (Carpenter & Buchanan, 1994). However, medication does not necessarily prevent relapse; even when individuals are receiving closely monitored antipsychotic medication, as many as 15-20% experience an increase in psychotic symptoms when followed for a one-year period (Kane & McGlashan, 1995). While dosing guidelines do not differ by gender, it has been observed that women with schizophrenia need lower doses than men and that, as a group, women have a somewhat better response to antipsychotic medication than men (Seeman, 2004). However, gender differences in dose response and treatment response appear to dissipate with advancing age (Canuso et al., 1998).

Based on the hypothesized role of estrogen as a protective factor in schizophrenia etiology, several small trials of estrogen as an adjunctive treatment for psychotic symptoms in premenopausal women with schizophrenia have been performed (Kulkarni et al., 2002; Akhondzadeh et al., 2003; Louza et al., 2004; Bergemann et al., 2005). Results of these studies have been mixed in terms of the efficacy of estrogen treatment and further studies are underway. At the current time, the use of estrogen as a treatment for schizophrenia is experimental.

Treatment recommendations for schizophrenia include specific psychosocial treatments including family education, skills training, and supported employment. These interventions have a strong evidence base but are not provided for most patients with schizophrenia in typical clinical settings (Lehman & Steinwachs, 1998). Given relatively low utilization of psychiatric services among older patients in general (Jin et al., 2003), it is likely that older persons with schizophrenia are even less likely to receive recommended treatments than younger ones. Of note, there are no specialized treatment guidelines or recommendations for older individuals, or older women, with schizophrenia. Several programs have been developed specifically for older individuals with schizophrenia that take into account the life issues of older individuals that may differ from those of younger persons, but these programs have not been widely disseminated (e.g., Granholm et al., 2005).

In the past, elderly persons with schizophrenia constituted a large proportion of individuals in public psychiatric hospitals. The locus of treatment has changed markedly and now about 85% of older individuals with schizophrenia reside in outpatient, community settings (Cohen et al., 2000). While some of these persons live independently, older individuals with schizophrenia are disproportionately represented in board and care residences, in adult foster care, and among the homeless. Based on previous studies showing that fewer than 50% of patients with schizophrenia in the community actually receive psychiatric care, one can assume that many older women with schizophrenia do not receive any psychiatric treatment (Von Korff et al., 1985).

Older women, as other patients with schizophrenia, are vulnerable to substandard living conditions and poverty. Older women with schizophrenia may also lack kinship ties and a strong personal support network that is an essential component of psychiatric care and treatment. Such women are also at risk for neglect of their physical health problems, problems which intensify with the aging process. As a group, individuals with schizophrenia have high rates of smoking, obesity, and other poor health behaviors and these problems are found, as well, in older women with the illness. Such women may also be less likely to receive routine medical care, such as mammography, than women in the general population (Dickerson et al., 2002).

CONCLUSIONS

Schizophrenia typically represents a lifelong and serious psychiatric disorder which persists into older years. Despite the fact that 1.6 million persons in America have schizophrenia, knowledge of the epidemiology of the disorder, especially in the later adult years, is limited. With changes in the age structure of the US population and increasing numbers of persons in older age groups, such knowledge is even more important in order to address the clinical needs of older patients.

While younger women with schizophrenia have a better prognosis than male patients, this gender advantage is less evident in older age groups. Older women with schizophrenia are vulnerable to problems of both schizophrenia and aging. Schizophrenia symptoms typically continue in later years and include ongoing psychotic symptoms and associated problems related to mood and life trauma. Problems of aging such as cognitive decline and chronic medical conditions may be exacerbated by schizophrenia. Such women are at risk for neglect of psychiatric and other health needs that are further compounded by limited social support and low socioeconomic status. The concept of "recovery" has been widely disseminated among younger patients with schizophrenia, but only limited attention has been given to a recovery model specifically developed for older individuals with the disorder. More research and clinical attention are needed to the problems of older women with schizophrenia.

REFERENCES

Akhondzadeh, S., Nejatisafa, A. A., Amini, H., Mohammadi, M. R., Larijani, B., Kashani, L., Raisi, F., & Kamalipour, A. (2003). Adjunctive estrogen treatment in women with chronic schizophrenia: A double-blind, randomized, and placebo-controlled trial. *Progress in Neuropsychopharmacology and Biological Psychiatry. 27,* 1007-1012.

American Psychiatric Association (APA) (1994). *Diagnostic and statistical manual of mental disorders* (DSM-IV) (4th Ed.). Washington, DC: American Psychiatric Press.

Bardenstein, K. K., & McGlashan, T. H. (1990). Gender differences in affective, schizo-affective, and schizophrenic disorders: A review. *Schizophrenia Research, 3,* 159-72.

Bergemann, N., Mundt, C., Parzer, P., Pakrasi, M., Eckstein-Mannsperger, U., Haisch, S., Salbach, B., Klinga, K., Runnebaum, B., & Resch, F. (2005). Estrogen as an adjuvant therapy to antipsychotics does not prevent relapse in women suffering from schizophrenia: Results of a placebo-controlled double-blind study. *Schizophrenia Research, 74,* 125-34.

Brown, S. (1997). Excess mortality of schizophrenia: A meta-analysis. *British Journal of Psychiatry, 171,* 502-508.

Canuso, C. M., Goldstein, J. M., & Green, A. I. (1998). The evaluation of women with schizophrenia. *Psychopharmacology Bulletin. 34,* 271-277.

Carpenter, W. T., & Buchanan, R W. (1994). Schizophrenia. *New England Journal of Medicine, 330,* 681-690.

Cohen, C. I., Cohen, G. D., Blank, K., Gaitz, C., Katz, I. R., Leuchter, A., Maletta, G., Meyers, B., Sakauye, K., & Shamoian, C. (2000). Schizophrenia and older adults. An overview: Directions for research and policy. *American Journal of Geriatric Psychiatry, 8,* 19-20.

Dickerson, F. B., Brown, C. H., Kreyenbuhl, J., Goldberg, R. W., Fang, L. J., & Dixon, L. B. (2004). Sexual and reproductive behaviors among persons with mental illness. *Psychiatric Services, 55,* 1299-1301.

Dickerson, F. B., Pater, A., & Origoni, A. E. (2002). Health behaviors and health status of older women with schizophrenia. *Psychiatric Services, 53,* 882-884.

Granholm, E., McQuaid, J. R., McClure, F. S., Auslander, L. A., Perivoliotis, D., Pedrelli, P., Patterson, T., & Jeste, D. V. (2005). A randomized, controlled trial of cognitive behavioral social skills training for middle-aged and older outpatients with chronic schizophrenia. *American Journal of Psychiatry, 162,* 520-529.

Harding, C. M., Brooks, G. W., Ashikaga, T., Strauss, J. S., & Breier, A. (1987). The Vermont longitudinal study of persons with severe mental illness, II: Long-term outcome of subjects who retrospectively met DSM-III criteria for schizophrenia. *American Journal of Psychiatry, 144,* 727-735.

Harris, M. J., & Jeste, D. V. (1988). Late-onset schizophrenia: An overview. *Schizophrenia Bulletin, 14,* 39-55.

Harvey, P. D., Silverman, J. M., Mohs, R. C., Parrella, M., White, L., Powchik, P., Davidson, M., & Davis, K. L. (1999). Cognitive decline in late-life schizophrenia: A longitudinal study of geriatric chronically hospitalized patients. *Biological Psychiatry, 45,* 32-40.

Hegarty, J. D., Baldessarini, R. J., Tohen, M., Waternaux, C., & Oepen, G. (1994). One hundred years of schizophrenia: A meta-analysis of the outcome literature. *American Journal of Psychiatry, 151,* 1409-1416.

Howard, R., Rabins, P. V., Seeman, M. V., & Jeste, D. V. (2000). Late-onset schizophrenia and very-late-onset schizophrenia-like psychosis: An international consensus. The International Late-Onset Schizophrenia Group. *American Journal of Psychiatry, 157,* 172-178.

Jeste, D. V., Twamley, E. W., Eyler-Zorrilla, L. T., Golshan, S., Patterson, T. L., & Palmer, B. W. (2003). Aging and outcome in schizophrenia. *Acta Psychiatrica Scandinavica, 107,* 336-343.

Jin, H., Folsom, D. P., Lindamer, L., Bailey, A., Hawthorne, W., Garcia, P., & Jeste, D. V. (2003). Patterns of public mental health service use by age in patients with schizophrenia. *American Journal of Geriatric Psychiatry, 5,* 525-533.

Kane, J. M., & McGlashan, T. H. (1995). Treatment of schizophrenia. *Lancet, 346,* 820-825.

Kessler, R. C., McGonagle, K. A., Zhao, S., Nelson, C. B., Hughes, M., Eshleman, S., Wittchen, H. U., & Kendler, K. S. (1994). Lifetime and 12-month prevalence of DSM-III-R psychiatric disorders in the United States: Results from the National Comorbidity Survey. *Archives of General Psychiatry, 51,* 8-19.

Kulkarni, J., Riedel, A., de Castella, A. R., Fitzgerald, P. B., Rolfe, T. J., Taffe, J., & Burger, H. (2002). A clinical trial of adjunctive estrogen treatment in women with schizophrenia. *Archives of Women and Mental Health, 5,* 99-104.

Lehman, A. F., Kreyenbuhl, J., Buchanan, R. W., Dickerson, F. B., Dixon, L. B., Goldberg, R., Green-Paden, L. D., Tenhula, W. N., Boerescu, D., Tek, C., Sandson, N., & Steinwachs, D. M. (2004). The Schizophrenia Patient Outcomes Research Team (PORT): Updated treatment recommendations. *Schizophrenia Bulletin. 30*, 193-217.

Lehman, A. F., & Steinwachs, D. M. (1998). Patterns of usual care for schizophrenia: Initial results from the Schizophrenia Patient Outcomes Research Team (PORT) Client Survey. *Schizophrenia Bulletin, 24*, 11-20.

Lehmann, S. W. (2003). Psychiatric disorders in older women. *International Review of Psychiatry, 15*, 269-279.

Leweke, F. M., Gerth, C. W., Koethe, D., Klosterkotter, J., Ruslanova, I., Krivogorsky, B., Torrey, E. F., & Yolken, R. H. (2004). Antibodies to infectious agents in individuals with recent onset schizophrenia. *European Archives of Psychiatry and Clinical Neuroscience, 254*, 4-8.

Lindamer, L. A., Lohr, J. B., Harris, M. J., McAdams, L. A., & Jeste, D. V. (1999). Gender-related clinical differences in older patients with schizophrenia. *Journal of Clinical Psychiatry, 60*, 61-67.

Louza, M. R., Marques, A. P., Elkis, H., Bassitt, D., Diegoli, M., & Gattaz, W. F. (2004). Estrogens as adjuvant therapy in the treatment of acute schizophrenia: A double-blind study. *Schizophrenia Research, 66*, 97-100.

Miller, L. J. (1997). Sexuality, reproduction, and family planning in women with schizophrenia. *Schizophrenia Bulletin, 23*, 623-635.

Miller, L. J., & Finnerty, M. (1996). Sexuality, pregnancy, and childrearing among women with schizophrenia-spectrum disorders. *Psychiatric Services, 47*, 502-506.

Mueser, K. T., & McGurk, S. R. (2004). Schizophrenia. *Lancet, 363*, 2063-2072.

Sajatovic, M., Sultana, D., Bingham, C. R., Buckley, P., & Donenwirth, K. (2002). Gender related differences in clinical characteristics and hospital based resource utilization among older adults with schizophrenia. *International Journal of Geriatric Psychiatry, 17*, 542-548.

Sawa, A., & Snyder, S. H. (2002). Schizophrenia: Diverse approaches to a complex disease. *Science, 296*, 692-695.

Seeman, M. V. (2004). Gender differences in the prescribing of antipsychotic drugs. *American Journal of Psychiatry, 161*, 1324-1333.

Sokal, J., Messias, E., Dickerson, F. B., Kreyenbuhl, J., Brown, C. H., Goldberg, R. W., & Dixon, L. B. (2004). Comorbidity of medical illnesses among adults with serious mental illness who are receiving community psychiatric services. *Journal of Nervous and Mental Disease, 2*, 421-427.

Torrey, E. F. (1992). Are we overestimating the genetic contribution to schizophrenia? *Schizophrenia Bulletin, 18*, 159-170.

Torrey, E. F. (2001). *Surviving schizophrenia*. New York: Harper Collins.

Von Korff, M., Nestadt, G., Romanoski, A., Anthony, J., Eaton, W., Merchant, A., Chahal, R., Kramer, M., Folstein, M., & Gruenberg, E. (1985). Prevalence of treated and untreated DSM-III Schizophrenia: Results of a two-stage community survey. *Journal of Nervous and Mental Disease, 173*, 577-581.

Yolken, R. H., & Torrey, E. F. (1995). Viruses, schizophrenia, and bipolar disorder. *Clinical Microbiol Review, 8*, 131-45.

doi:10.1300/J074v19n01_04

Major Depressive Disorder
in the Older Adult:
Implications for Women

Reed D. Goldstein, PhD
Alan M. Gruenberg, MD

SUMMARY. Mood disorders manifest across the life span yet often go undiagnosed and untreated. Increasingly, Major Depressive Disorder (MDD) in the older adult is recognized as a frequently occurring, heterogeneous psychiatric illness that impacts the individual and family, one's physical health, and society. Women are more likely to be diagnosed with MDD than men and therefore it is important to identify specific risk factors and other distinguishing features. This article reviews the descriptive characteristics, epidemiology, etiology and pathophysiology, course and natural history, and assessment and treatment of MDD with specific focus on women and aging. doi:10.1300/J074v19n01_05 *[Article copies available for a fee from The Haworth Document Delivery Service: 1-800-HAWORTH. E-mail address: <docdelivery@haworthpress.com> Website: <http://www.HaworthPress.com> © 2007 by The Haworth Press, Inc. All rights reserved.]*

KEYWORDS. Depression, women, aging, mood disorders, dysthymia

---

Address correspondence to: Reed D. Goldstein, 245 S. 8th Street, Office 140, Philadelphia, PA 19107 (E-mail: Goldster@pahosp.com).

[Haworth co-indexing entry note]: "Major Depressive Disorder in the Older Adult: Implications for Women." Goldstein, Reed D., and Alan M. Gruenberg. Co-published simultaneously in *Journal of Women & Aging* (The Haworth Press, Inc.) Vol. 19, No. 1/2, 2007, pp. 63-78; and: *Mental Health Issues of Older Women: A Comprehensive Review for Health Care Professionals* (ed: Victor J. Malatesta) The Haworth Press, Inc., 2007, pp. 63-78. Single or multiple copies of this article are available for a fee from The Haworth Document Delivery Service [1-800-HAWORTH, 9:00 a.m. - 5:00 p.m. (EST). E-mail address: docdelivery@haworthpress.com].

Available online at http://jwa.haworthpress.com
© 2007 by The Haworth Press, Inc. All rights reserved.
doi:10.1300/J074v19n01_05

INTRODUCTION AND DEFINITION
OF DEPRESSIVE DISORDERS

Depressive disorders have plagued mankind since the earliest documentation of human experience. Major depressive disorder (MDD), dysthymic disorder (DD), and depressive disorder not otherwise specified (DDNOS) are the group of clinical conditions in the Diagnostic and Statistical Manual of Mental Disorders, Fourth Edition–Text Revision (DSM- IV-TR; American Psychiatric Association, 2000) characterized by depressive symptomatology. These conditions specifically exclude a history of manic, mixed or hypomanic episodes, and are not due to the physiologic effects of substances of abuse, other medications, or toxins. In the longitudinal course, an individual may suffer from both DD and MDD, referred to as double depression (Keller & Shapiro, 1982).

All of these depressive disorders require prospective observation because subsequent symptoms such as mania or psychosis can result in a change in diagnosis. For example, when an episode of depression remits and is subsequently followed by a manic episode, the diagnosis is changed from MDD to bipolar disorder. When DD evolves into MDD, and the patient subsequently develops an episode of hypomania, re-diagnosis of the condition to bipolar II disorder is required.

The depressive disorders are characterized by lifelong vulnerability to episodes of disease, involving depressed mood or loss of interest and pleasure in activities. Typically, a distinction is drawn between a feeling state of dejection, sadness, or unhappiness, which may be brief in duration, and a clinical syndrome characterized by persistent sadness, profound discouragement, or despair which persists two weeks or more and is associated with a change from previous functioning. Changes in mood are experienced by an individual as a feeling of sadness, irritability, dejection, despair, or loss of interest or pleasure. Neurovegetative or biological signs of depression include impairment in sleep, appetite, energy level, libido, and psychomotor activity. Prominent symptoms also include marked impairment in concentration with increased distractibility, and the presence of guilty preoccupation.

Beck (1973) emphasized cognitive manifestations of depression, including distortions about oneself, one's experience in the world and the future, accompanied by self-blame and indecision. These core symptoms of depression are evident in children or adolescents with MDD although the depressed mood may be manifested by irritability or social withdrawal. In contrast, older adults show a preponderance of somatic preoccupation and memory impairment.

Current definitions of MDD emphasize suicidal ideation, thoughts of death, and suicide attempts as a cardinal criterion symptom of the disorder. Suicidality is the feature of depressive disorder that poses substantial risk of mortality in the disease. Prevention of suicide, more than any other treatment goal, requires immediate intervention and may require hospitalization. The risk for subsequent completed suicide for an individual hospitalized for an episode of severe MDD is estimated to be at 15% (Coryell et al., 1982).

EPIDEMIOLOGY

The literature reflects that the prevalence and incidence data on MDD vary to some degree due to methodological differences, nature of interview format, geographic location, and setting of sample. Large-scale epidemiologic studies of mood disorders began in the 1950s, culminating with a reanalysis of the NIMH epidemiologic catchment area (ECA; Weissman et al., 1988) study, and more recently, results from the National Comorbidity Survey (NCS; Kessler et al., 1994).

Across epidemiologic studies, MDD is identified as a common psychiatric disorder throughout the life span, and is often characterized by gender differences. The lifetime risk for MDD in community samples varies from 10 to 25% for women and 5 to 12% for men (American Psychiatric Association, 2000). The point prevalence of MDD for adults in community samples has varied from 5 to 9% for women and from 2 to 3% for men (American Psychiatric Association, 2000). Notably, while the incidence rates of MDD in prepubertal boys and girls are equal, women over the course of their lifetime are two to three times more likely to have MDD after puberty (Kornstein, 1997).

A strong relationship exists between low social class and schizophrenia whereas a weaker but nevertheless meaningful relationship may exist between low income status and the occurrence of MDD. Analyses of the ECA data indicated that the lowest income group manifested twice the risk of MDD than the highest income group, while the NCS concluded that individuals with low socioeconomic status demonstrate higher risk for MDD than individuals who are economically well-off. Rates of MDD may also be influenced by low-income status (Blazer et al., 1994) as well as childhood adversity including severe physical abuse, sexual abuse, and neglect (Harkness & Monroe, 2002).

Lifetime risk refers to the proportion of individuals being studied who would go on to develop the disorder during their lifetime. Estimates of lifetime risk of MDD in community samples vary from 20 to 25% for women and 7 to 12% for men (Depression Guideline Panel, 1993). Lifetime prevalence refers to those individuals who, up to the time of assessment, have had symptoms that met diagnostic criteria at some point in their lives. The NCS estimated overall lifetime prevalence of MDD as 17.1%. The estimated prevalence was twice as high in females than males. Point prevalence or current prevalence refers to the proportion of the individuals who have the disorder being studied at a designated time (Boyd & Weismann, 1981). The specific point prevalence of MDD in community samples has ranged from 5 to 9% for women and 2 to 3% for men. The point prevalence of MDD in primary care outpatient setting ranges from 4.8 to 8.6% (Depression Guideline Panel, 1993). In hospitalized medical patients, more than 14% had MDD (Feldman et al., 1987).

Epidemiologic studies have focused on the older adult population as well. Weissman and colleagues (1991) found a 1% prevalence of MDD in adults 65 years and older who lived in the community, and 2.3% of women 65 and older met criteria for dysthymia. The data indicate that a lower lifetime prevalence of MDD was found in the oldest age group ($\geq$ age 65) in comparison to younger age groups. Women manifest an increased prevalence of MDD in comparison to men, and no significant differences were found across racial or ethnic groups. However, other community samples of older adults were found to have a high prevalence (8-15%) of clinically significant depressive symptoms (but not a formal diagnosis of MDD). In comparison to community settings, higher prevalence rates for MDD are found in treatment settings for older adults: 11% in hospitals, 5% in outpatient nonpsychiatric clinics, and 12% in long-term care settings (Blazer, 1994).

In her review, Nolen-Hoeksema (1987) noted that the higher prevalence of depression in women relative to men was found in various regions of the world regardless of diagnostic and interview method. Weissman et al. (1993) raised the possibility that the rates of depression expressed by both genders was growing closer, however. More recent studies have suggested that older women manifest lower rates of MDD in comparison to younger women (Jeste et al., 1999), and that the greater prevalence of MDD in women relative to men diminishes somewhat with increasing age (Barefoot et al., 2001). Rokke and Klenow (1998) considered that rates of depression in men could remain stable or increase during the life span whereas women could have decreasing rates of depression thereby explaining the more similar rates of depression in older adult males and females. Men who live alone or outlive their spouses are particularly vulnerable to depression. Women may be more resilient in later life, if widowed or living alone.

Risk Factors

Depression is known to impact on the workplace setting and economy, time spent in leisure activities, and social relationships. The Global Burden of Disease study (Murray & Lopez, 1996) reported that unipolar major depression was the main source of disease-related disability for females throughout the world for ages five years and older. The Depression Guideline Panel (1993) presented 10 risk factors for depression: (1) history of prior episodes; (2) family history of depressive disorder especially in first-degree relatives; (3) history of suicide attempts; (4) female gender; (5) age of onset before age 40; (6) postpartum period; (7) comorbid medical illness; (8) absence of social support; (9) negative, stressful life events; (10) active alcohol or substance abuse.

Whereas a 4 to 5% current prevalence rate of MDD exists in community samples, symptoms of depression are found in 12 to 36% of patients with a general medical condition (Depression Guideline Panel, 1993). The rate of depression may be higher in patients with a specific medical condition, a finding relevant to the older adult. MDD is identified as an independent condition and calls for specific treatment when it occurs in the presence of a general medical condition.

For example, some post-stroke older adult patients manifest depression due to cerebrovascular disease related to cerebral infarction in left frontal and left subcortical brain regions. A point prevalence of mood disorder due to cerebrovascular disease in post-stroke patients between 10 and 27% has been documented, with an average duration of depression lasting approximately one year (Depression Guideline Panel, 1993) characterized by poor treatment compliance, irritability, and personality change (Ross & Rush, 1981). The issue of dementia and the older adult is addressed elsewhere in this volume, and the distinction between depressive disorders and dementing disorders is often complicated because depression and dementia commonly co-occur. Treatment of co-occurring depressive features may relieve symptoms and improve overall quality of life.

Approximately 50% of patients with Parkinson's disease experience a MDD during course of illness. Treatment of the depressive disorder may result in improvement in the signs and symptoms of depression without alleviation of the involuntary movement disorder or cognitive changes associated with subcortical brain disease. The underlying etiology of associated dementia and depressive disorder in Parkinson's disease appears to involve physiologic changes in subcortical brain regions. The older adult with medical conditions including, but not necessarily limited to, diabetes, coronary artery disease, or cancer must be carefully monitored as a high prevalence of depression is identified in those individuals.

Gruenberg and Goldstein (2003) reviewed comorbidity patterns of MDD and other clinical psychiatric disorders such as alcohol/drug dependence, anxiety disorders, obsessive-compulsive disorder, post-traumatic stress disorder, somatization disorder, eating disorders and personality disorders. More than 40% of patients with MDD have additional symptoms that meet criteria during their lifetime for one or more additional psychiatric disorders (Sargeant et al., 1990). The presence of a comorbid psychiatric disorder may alter the course of major mood disorder in a dramatic fashion and is identified as a primary risk factor for poor treatment response. Specific guidelines are available to inform decision-making regarding which illness (MDD or other psychiatric disorder) becomes the initial focus of treatment (Depression Guideline Panel, 1993).

Other risk factors have been considered. Kessler and McLeod (1984) found that men became more depressed than women in response to financial strain whereas women became more depressed in response to family problems. Recently, Kessler (2003) reported that women have a higher risk than men of first onset which accounts for the gender differences in the prevalence of depression, while there is less evidence in support of gender differences in recurrent or chronic depression. Furthermore, Gatz and Fiske (2003) stated that being an older woman per se does not increase the risk for MDD. Kessler (2003) reviewed identified risk factors for women, and argued that the interaction of biological factors or vulnerabilities (e.g., changes in sex hormones) with environmental factors was most likely to eventually explain gender differences in depression.

ETIOLOGY AND PATHOPHYSIOLOGY

Greater understanding of the underlying etiology and pathophysiology of MDD is the focus of genetic, neurobiologic, and psychosocial investigation. Kendler et al. (1992) estimated a 33 to 45% genetic liability to depression in women depending on the criteria used to diagnose MDD.

Moreover, a moderate role for individual specific environmental experiences was demonstrated to influence the risk for depression. Given the estimated heritability in MDD, converging evidence supports the important role of environmental experiences in the etiology of major depression (Brown & Harris, 1978).

Gruenberg and Goldstein (2003) reviewed neurobiological theories of depression. The range of neurobiological changes associated with depression and the elderly may include alterations in a number hypothalamic-pituitary axis functions. This includes impact of cortisol changes within the hypothalamic-pituitary-adrenal axis. A very consistent finding across all ages but particularly evident in older adults with depression is elevated cortisol. This finding is also part of the understanding of external stress and stress-related dysfunction in those who develop depression. Anatomical changes have been associated with late onset depression, including reduced volume of the hippocampus, reduced volume in the prefrontal cortex, and reduced volume in the anterior cingulate, caudate and amygdala.

There are associated neuroendocrine axis abnormalities associated with depression in the elderly including mild increases in TSH and anti-thyroid antibody formation as well as mild blunting of TSH response which places elderly women at risk for further bone loss, cognitive dysfunction, and depression. In women, menopause is associated with an evolution of estrogen deficiency. The presence of postmenopausal estrogen depletion has been associated with vasomotor symptoms, urogenital changes, atrophy, decreased cognition and greater vulnerability to major depressive disorder (MDD) as well as dysthymia and even dysphoria in the setting of physical illness and other stressful life events. The examination of depression in the elderly shows similar hypothalamic-pituitary-adrenal axis abnormalities as seen in younger adults with serious depressive disorders and significantly different from non-depressed elderly controls (Seidman, 2004).

Psychoanalytic theory (Abraham, 1927; Freud, 1957) addressed the role of urges, conflicts, and their resolution. Freud asserted that periodic depression and melancholia appeared in combination with severe anxiety. He emphasized the common ground between neurasthenia and melancholia, noting that neurasthenic symptoms characterized by prominent anxiety were often accompanied by depression, an observation that set the stage for psychiatry's current focus on comorbid syndromal clinical presentations. Also, Freud and Abraham emphasized the connection between mourning and melancholia, through the introjection and identification with an ambivalently-experienced lost object. The melancholic patient experiences a loss of self-esteem with associated hopelessness and helplessness, prominent guilt, and self-denigration, resulting from internally directed anger. Anger or aggression associated with ambivalence is turned against the self, leading to the depressive experience. Gruenberg and Goldstein (2003) summarized other psychoanalytic contributions. Recent trauma theories emphasize the distinction between global self-esteem and an experience of self, which has been altered by past traumatic experiences. This duality of self may persist into later years in women, making them vulnerable to depression when exposed to loss.

The behavioral perspective focuses on an overgeneralized depressive response to loss of social support. The individual's social environment no longer provides reinforcement, and the depressed patient comes to feel isolated and unsupported. The lack of social support appears to be one of the strongest factors in promoting vulnerability to depression (Skinner, 1953). Furthermore, the experience of depression elicits negative responses from others, including rejection from spouses, children, or other important individuals. Coyne (1976) noted that the persistence of depression is associated with the continuing experience of negative responses from others. Lewinsohn (1974) suggested that individuals with depression have social skills deficits that make it difficult to obtain reinforcement from the social environment.

The cognitive-behavioral theory is the most empirically examined psychosocial theory in relation to the management and treatment of the depressed patient. The cognitive-behavioral perspective originally developed by Beck (1976) emphasizes a set of dysfunctional attitudes, cognitions, and images associated with depressive symptomatology. Beck posited that cognitive distortions cause depression and are associated with maintenance of the disorder. The "cognitive triad" involves negative views of one's self, one's world and current situation, and the future. Also, the cognitive theory delineates the importance of cognitive distortions, the "cognitive triad," and a conception of negative self-image which is called negative self-schemas. The cognitive perspective is elaborated further by learned helplessness models, and hopelessness theory (Abramson, 1989; Seligman, 1975).

In cognitive-behavioral therapy (CBT; Beck, 1973), education, behavioral assignments, and cognitive retraining form the active components of psychotherapy (Beck et al., 1979). This cognitive therapy has been demonstrated to be an effective short-term psychotherapy for depression (DeRubeis et al., 1990).

The current iteration of an interpersonal approach is reflected in the development of a specific treatment for depression termed interpersonal psychotherapy of depression (IPT) (Klerman et al., 1984). IPT involves a formal diagnostic assessment, inventory of important current and past relationships, and definition of the current problem area. In IPT, four areas of focus that could relate to depressive symptoms are: (1) grief; (2) interpersonal role disputes; (3) role transitions; and (4) interpersonal deficits.

Social rhythm theory focuses on the disruption of biological rhythms associated with psychosocial stressors. The loss of "social zeitgebers" has been proposed as a link between biological and psychosocial formulations (Ehlers, 1988). The social zeitgebers theory suggests that social relationships, interpersonal continuity, and work tasks entrain biological rhythms. Disruptions of social rhythms due to loss of relationships interfere with biological rhythms that maintain homeostasis. This disruption leads to changes in neurobiological processes including alterations in neurotransmitter functions, neuroendocrine regulation, and neuorophysiologic control of sleep/wake cycle and other normal circadian oscillations.

Other factors could explain the etiology of depression in women and the different rates of depression in males and females. Mirowsky and Ross (1989) offered that the traditional female role is associated with significant and chronic stress, which subsequently results in higher rates of depression in women than men. Also, women were found to brood or worry about problems more than men, and therefore temporary or transient upset or symptoms of dysphoria evolve into an episode of MDD ("rumination theory"; Nolen-Hoeksema, 1990).

COURSE AND NATURAL HISTORY

The mean age of onset of major depression is 27 years of age (Weissman et al., 1988), although an individual can experience the onset of MDD at any age. New symptoms of MDD tend to develop over several days to several weeks. Early manifestations of an episode of MDD include anxiety, sleeplessness, worry, and rumination prior to the experience of overt depression. Over a lifetime, the presence of one major depressive episode is associated with a 50% chance of a recurrent episode (Thase, 1990). A history of two episodes is associated with a 70 to 80% risk of a future episode. Three or more episodes are associated with extremely high rates of recurrence. Individuals with recurrent episodes of depression are at greater risk to manifest bipolar disorder (Depression Guideline Panel, 1993). Because the majority of cases of MDD recur, continuation treatment and ongoing education regarding warning signs of relapse or recurrence are essential in ongoing clinical care.

Untreated episodes of depression last six to 24 months (Goodwin & Jamison, 1990). Symptom remission and a return to premorbid level of functioning characterize approximately 66% of depressed patients (Depression Guideline Panel, 1993). By comparison, approximately 5 to 10% of patients continue to experience a full episode of depression for greater than two years, and approximately 20 to 25% of patients experience only partial recovery between episodes. Furthermore, 25% manifest "double depression," characterized by the development of MDD superimposed upon a mild chronic DD (Keller & Shapriro, 1982). Patients with double depression often demonstrate poor inter-episode recovery.

Older adults with depression tend to report more somatic symptoms than affective symptoms, and complain of loss of interest, pleasure and emotion while denying change in mood (Gallo & Rabins, 1999). Often, older adults experience cognitive impairment as part of the clinical syndrome. Symptoms of depression may simulate dementia with concentration difficulties, memory loss, and distractibility. Comorbid medical conditions impact on the course of depression in older adults as well.

Roughly 50% of older adults experience their first episode of depression in the latter part of life. Consideration of medical and psychosocial factors (e.g., retirement or loss of spouse) is necessary when addressing the course of MDD in the older adult. Perimenopausal women are likely to acknowledge depressive symptoms such as labile mood, diminished energy, and absence of motivation (Steiner et al., 2003).

Finally, the clinician must assess the patient's level of suicidality throughout the course of illness. Conwell (2004) noted that the rates of completed suicide are highest later in life. In the United States, the highest-risk group is thought to be old white males, and the highest-risk period for women is midlife.

ASSESSMENT AND TREATMENT

The assessment of MDD involves identification of five of nine criterion symptoms (DSM-IV-TR; American Psychiatric Association, 2000). The clinician undertakes a medical assessment, evaluates for presence of comorbid psychiatric disorders, obtains family history, assesses risk for suicide, and learns about significant life events in order to provide effective treatment to the depressed older adult. Gruenberg and Goldstein (2003) reviewed relevant laboratory studies, neuropsychological tests, and symptom severity rating scales.

The new onset of psychiatric disorder in an adult 65 or older requires the careful consideration of medical, social, and psychological issues. Concurrent medication treatment of primary medical conditions may cause psychiatric symptoms in the elderly. Therefore, among the medical diseases which affect the older adults, one must evaluate the consequences of vascular changes due to coronary artery diseases, hypertension, and cerebrovascular disease. The assessment requires understanding of the effects of inflammation due to arthritis or other rheumatoid illnesses. One must also assess the effects of traumatic physical injuries. In the context of new onset depression and weight loss, one must consider the presence of neoplasm or cancer.

Any age-related change in the brain or other organ systems will affect how the person tolerates specific medications. The clinician must understand the mechanism of action and side effects of every medication taken by the older patient, including over-the-counter sleep or pain medications.

Many new onset episodes of depression in the elderly are due to another neurological or neurodegenerative disease such as Dementia of the Alzheimer's Type, multiple infarcts or certain subcortical vascular changes consistent with vascular depression, or neurological conditions such as Parkinson's Disease.

Specific depression-based psychological treatment for MDD is available (Gruenberg & Goldstein, 2003). These treatments have included supportive psychiatric management techniques during pharmacotherapy, interpersonal psychotherapy, cognitive-behavioral therapy, brief dynamic psychotherapy, and marital and family therapy. Psychiatric management and supportive therapy is the standard in psychiatric office practice, and is characterized by establishing a positive therapeutic relationship in the course of diagnosis and initiation of treatment of depression, provision of education, collaboration with the patient, and supportive feedback. The supportive psychotherapeutic management of depression facilitates the pharmacologic response.

Interpersonal psychotherapy of depression (IPT), which is demonstrated to be effective in acute treatment trials (Elkin et al., 1989), addresses interpersonal difficulties such as interpersonal loss or grieving, role transitions, interpersonal disputes, and social deficits. The depressed female older adult, who could be struggling with loss of spouse or change in marital status, or transition from workplace to retirement or from having raised a family to an empty home, benefits from IPT.

Cognitive-behavioral therapy (CBT) for depression reduces symptoms through the identification and correction of cognitive distortions. Controlled studies have demonstrated the efficacy of cognitive therapy in resolution of MDD in adults (Depression Guideline Panel, 1993). IPT or CBT is effective in the treatment of mild depression. However, medication treatment is associated with the most rapid response, and is superior to both interpersonal psychotherapy and cognitive-behavioral psychotherapy in more severely depressed patients.

Brief dynamic psychotherapy, which was not specifically designed for treatment of MDD, addresses current conflicts as manifestations of difficulty in early attachment. Similarly, research is needed to determine the efficacy of marital and family therapy in individuals with MDD. However, marital distress is a major event associated with the development of a depressive episode, marital discord often will persist after the remission of depression, and subsequent relapses are frequently associated with disruptions of marital relationships.

For the pharmacologic treatment of late life depression, principles associated with antidepressant treatment include a slower rate of response and slightly decreased overall rate of response to antidepressant medications. The older adult may require a more extended treatment trial, and the clinician must focus on the emergence of any adverse side effects which may occur.

The most common antidepressants offered to the older adult are standard selective serotonin reuptake inhibitors (SSRIs) including citalopram (Celexa), escitalopram (Lexapro), and sertraline (Zoloft). Other antidepressants are considered dual serotonin and norepinephrine reuptake inhibitors (SNRIs) such as venlafaxine (Effexor) and duloxetine (Cymbalta). In the setting of genetic or prior history of hypomania or mania, mood stabilizing medications are required such as lithium carbonate or anticonvulsants, used for prevention of episodes of mania or depression.

In the older adult with prominent fatigue and anhedonia, some clinicians may favor the use of buproprion (Wellbutrin), which has predominant norepinephrine and dopaminergic effects. The use of stimulants such as mixed amphetamine salts (Adderall) or methylphenidate (Ritalin) may be helpful. If the mood disorder is complicated by psychotic features, then standard dopamine inhibitors, either first or second generation, are required. If the mood disorder is associated with severe medical complications, malnutrition or dehydration, then a standard course of electroconvulsive therapy (ECT) may be life saving.

Any somatic treatment in the older adult is substantially augmented by regular exercise and consistent participation in structured social activities and personal relationships.

CONCLUSION

Depressive disorders in the older adult population, including women, are common, recurrent, and significantly impact quality of life. Treatment of any concurrent medical problems is warranted. In the presence of co-occurring depression, effective pharmacologic treatments are available, and psychotherapies systematically applied may achieve remission in depressive symptoms, resulting in improvement in the older adult's overall social, physical and interpersonal functioning.

REFERENCES

Abraham, K. (1927). Notes on the psychoanalytic investigation and treatment of manic-depressive insanity and allied conditions. In Institute of Psychoanalysis (Eds.), *Selected papers on psychoanalysis* (pp. 418-502). Hogarth Press: London.

Abramson, L. Y., Metalsky, G. I., & Alloy, L. B. (1989). Hopelessness depression: A theory-based subtype of depression. *Psychological Review, 96*, 358-372.

American Psychiatric Association (2000). *Diagnostic and statistical manual of mental disorders.* Fourth Edition. Text Revision, APA, Washington, DC.

Barefoot, J. C., Mortensen, E. L., Helms, M. J., Avlund, K., & Schroll, M. (2001). A longitudinal study of gender differences in depressive symptoms from age 50 to 80. *Psychology and Aging, 16*, 342-345.

Beck, A. T. (1973). *The diagnosis and management of depression.* University of Pennsylvania Press, Philadelphia.

Beck, A. T. (1976). *Cognitive therapy and the emotional disorders.* International University Press: New York.

Beck, A. T., Rush, A. J., & Shaw, B. F. (1979). *Cognitive therapy of depression.* Guilford Press: New York.

Blazer, D. G. (1994). Epidemiology of late-life depression. In L. S. Schneider & B. D. Lebowityz (Eds.), *Diagnosis and treatment of depression in late life: Results of the NIH Consensus Development Conference* (pp. 9-19). American Psychiatric Press: Washington, DC.

Blazer, D. G., Kessler, R. C., & McGonagle, K. A. (1994). The prevalence and distribution of major depression in a national comorbidity survey. *American Journal of Psychiatry, 151*, 979-986.

Boyd, J. H. & Weismann (1981). Epidemiology of affective disorders. *Archives of General Psychiatry, 38*, 1039-1046.

Brown, G. W. & Harris, T. (1978). *Social origins of depression: A study of psychiatric disorder in women*. Free Press: New York.

Conwell, Y. (2004). Suicide. In S. P. Roose & H. A. Sackeim (Eds.), *Late-life depression* (pp. 95-106). Oxford University Press.

Coryell, W. R., Noyes, R., & Clancy, J. (1982). Excess mortality in panic disorder: A comparison with primary unipolar depression. *Archives of General Psychiatry, 39*, 701-703.

Coyne, J. C. (1976). Toward an interactional description of depression. *Psychiatry, 39*, 28-40.

Depression Guideline Panel (1993). Depression in primary care: Vol. 1. *Detection and diagnosis, clinical practice guideline*, No. 5 (April). U.S. Department of Health and Human Services, Public Health Agency, Agency for Health Care and Policy Research. AHCPR Publication No. 93-0551.

DeRubeis, R. J., Hollon, S. D., Grove, W. M. et al. (1990). How does cognitive therapy work? Cognitive change and symptom in cognitive therapy and pharmacotherapy for depression. *Journal of Consulting and Clinical Psychiatry, 58* (6), 862-869.

Ehlers, C. L., Frank, E., & Kupfer, D. J. (1988). Social zeitgebers and biological rhythms. *Archives of General Psychiatry, 45*, 948-952.

Elkin, I., Shea, T. M., & Watkins, J. T. (1989). National Institute of Mental Health Treatment of Depression Collaborative Research Program. *Archives of General Psychiatry, 46*, 971-982.

Feldman, E., Hawton, M. R., & Arden, M. (1987). Psychiatric disorder in medical inpatients. *Q. Journal of Medicine, 63*, 405-412.

Freud, S. (1957). Mourning and melancholia. In J. Strachey (Trans-ed.), *The standard edition of the complete psychological works of Sigmund Freud*, Volume 14 (pp. 237-258). Hogarth Press: London.

Gallo, J. J. & Rabins, P. V. (1999). Depression without sadness: Alternative presentations of depression in late life. *American Family Physician, 60* (3), 820-826.

Gatz, M. & Fiske, A. (2003). *Professional Psychology: Research and Practice, 34* (1), 3-9.

Goodwin, F. K. & Jamison, K. R. (1990). *Manic-depressive illness*. Oxford University Press: New York.

Gruenberg, A. M. & Goldstein, R. D. (2003). Mood disorders: Depression. In A. Tasman, J. Kay, & J. A. Lieberman (Eds.), *Psychiatry*. Second Edition. Volume 2 (pp. 1207-1236). John Wiley & Sons, Ltd.

Harkness, K. L. & Monroe, S. M. (2002). Childhood adversity and the endogenous versus nonendogenous distinction in women with major depression. *American Journal of Psychiatry, 159*, 387-393.

Jeste, D. V., Alexopoulos, G. S., Baratels, S. J., Cummings, J. L., Gallo, J. J., Gottlied, G. L., et al. (1999). Consensus statement on the upcoming crisis in geriatric mental health. *Archives of General Psychiatry, 56*, 848-853.

Keller, M. B. & Shapiro, R.W. (1982). "Double depression": Superimposition of acute depressive episodes on chronic depressive disorders. *American Journal of Psychiatry, 139*, 438-442.

Kendler, K. S., Neale, M. C., & Kessler, R. C. (1992). A population-based twin study of major depression in women. *Archives of General Psychiatry, 49*, 257-266.

Kessler, R. C. (2003). Epidemiology of women and depression. *Journal of Affective Disorders, 74*, 5-13.

Kessler, R. C. & McLeod, J. D. (1984). Sex differences in vulnerability to undesirable life events. *American Sociological Review, 49*, 620-631.

Kessler, R. C., McGonagle, K. A., & Zhao, S. (1994). Lifetime and 12-month prevalence of DSM-III-R psychiatric disorders in United States. *Archives of General Psychiatry, 51*, 8-19.

Klerman, G. I., Weissman, M. M., & Rounsaville, B. J. (1984). *Interpersonal psychotherapy of depression.* Basic Books: New York.

Kornstein, S. G. (1997). Gender differences in depression: Implications for treatment. *Journal of Clinical Psychiatry, 58* (Supplement 15), 12-18.

Lewinsohn, P. M. (1974). A behavioral approach to depression. In R. J. Friedman & M. M. Katz (Eds.), *The psychology of depression: Contemporary theory and research.* John Wiley: New York.

Mirowsky, J. & Ross, C. E. (1989). *Social causes of psychological distress.* Aldine De Gruyter: New York.

Murray, C. J. L. & Lopez, A. D. (1996). Alternative visions of the future: Projecting mortality and disability, 1990-2020. In C. J. L. Murray & A. D. Lopez (Eds.), *The global burden of disease: A comprehensive assessment of mortality and disability from diseases, injuries, and risk factors in 1990 and projected to 2020* (pp. 325-395). Harvard University Press: Boston.

Nolen-Hoeksema, S. (1987). Sex differences in unipolar depression: Evidence and theory. *Psychological Bulletin, 101*, 259-282.

Nolen-Hoeksema, S. (1990). *Sex differences in depression.* Stanford University Press: Stanford, CA.

Rokke, P. D. & Klenow, D. J. (1998). Prevalence of depressive symptoms among rural elderly: Examining the need for mental health services. *Psychotherapy, 35*, 545-558.

Ross, E. D. & Rush, A. J. (1981). Diagnosis and neuroanatomical correlates of depression in brain-damaged patients: Implications for a neurology of depression. *Archives of General Psychiatry, 38*, 1344-1354.

Sargeant, J. K., Bruce, M. L., & Florio, L. P. (1990). Factors associated with 1-year outcome of major depression in the community. *Archives of General Psychiatry, 47*, 519-526.

Seidman, S. N. (2004). The neuroendocrinology of aging. In S. P. Roose & H. A. Sackeim (Eds.), *Late-life depression* (pp. 167-181). Oxford University Press.

Seligman, M. E. P. (1975). *Helplessness: On depression, development and death.* W. H. Freeman: San Francisco.

Skinner, B. F. (1953). *Science and human behavior.* Free Press: New York.

Steiner, M., Dunn, E., & Born, L. (2003). Hormones and mood: From menarche to menopause and beyond. *Journal of Affective Disorders, 74*, 67-83.

Thase, M. (1990). Relapse and recurrence in unipolar major depression: Short-term and long-term approaches. *Journal of Clinical Psychiatry, 51* (Supplement 6), 51-57.

Weissman, M. M., Bland, R., Joyce, P. R., & Newman, S. (1993). Sex differences in rates of depression: Cross-national perspectives (Special Issue: Toward a new psychobiology of depression in women). *Journal of Affective Disorders, 29* (2-3), 77-84.

Weissman, M. M., Bruce, M. L., & Leaf, P. J . (1991). Affective disorders. In L. N. Robins & D. A. Reiger (Eds.), *Psychiatric disorders in America* (pp. 53-80). Free Press: New York.

Weissman, M. M., Leaf, P. J., & Tischler, G. L. (1988). Affective disorders in five United States communities. *Psychological Medicine, 18,* 141-153.

doi:10.1300/J074v19n01_05

Anxiety Disorders and Older Women

Stephen Levine, PhD

Jay Weissman, PhD

SUMMARY. Anxiety is a problem for millions of Americans. It poses special challenges for women as they grow into advanced age. This paper provides a general overview of anxiety disorders, including panic disorder, agoraphobia, specific phobia, social phobia, obsessive compulsive disorder, and generalized anxiety disorder. Etiology, assessment and treatment strategies are then addressed. Special focus is directed at biological and psychosocial issues as they relate to older women in the development, experience, treatment and prevention of anxiety disorders. doi:10.1300/J074v19n01_06 *[Article copies available for a fee from The Haworth Document Delivery Service: 1-800-HAWORTH. E-mail address: <docdelivery@haworthpress.com> Website: <http://www.HaworthPress.com> © 2007 by The Haworth Press, Inc. All rights reserved.]*

KEYWORDS. Anxiety, women, aging, panic, phobia, obsessive compulsive disorder

INTRODUCTION

Anxiety disorders, which include symptoms of fear and worry, are one of the most commonly diagnosed psychiatric conditions in the

Address correspondence to: Stephen Levine, 741 Red Oak Terrace, Wayne, PA 19087.

[Haworth co-indexing entry note]: "Anxiety Disorders and Older Women." Levine, Stephen, and Jay Weissman. Co-published simultaneously in *Journal of Women & Aging* (The Haworth Press, Inc.) Vol. 19, No. 1/2, 2007, pp. 79-101; and: *Mental Health Issues of Older Women: A Comprehensive Review for Health Care Professionals* (ed: Victor J. Malatesta) The Haworth Press, Inc., 2007, pp. 79-101. Single or multiple copies of this article are available for a fee from The Haworth Document Delivery Service [1-800-HAWORTH, 9:00 a.m. - 5:00 p.m. (EST). E-mail address: docdelivery@haworthpress.com].

Available online at http://jwa.haworthpress.com
© 2007 by The Haworth Press, Inc. All rights reserved.
doi:10.1300/J074v19n01_06

United States (Craske, 2003). Lifetime prevalence rates for anxiety disorders are estimated to be 24.9%, and 17.2% for any 12-month period in the general population. Lifetime prevalence rates for females are estimated to be 30.5%, and 22.6% for any given 12-month period (Barlow, 2004). Among older women, the prevalence rate of those suffering from any type of anxiety disorder is estimated at 11.2% (Fisher et al., 2001). At nearly every age group, women are twice as likely as men to suffer from an anxiety disorder (Craske & Chowdhury, 2003; Zarit & Zarit, 1998).

Given the pattern of waxing and waning of symptoms over time, this suggests that current treatment strategies for many anxiety disorders are not completely effective. This presents a significant problem as anxiety disorders may cause considerable distress for individuals, including impairment in social and vocational functioning. If left untreated, anxiety disorders may play a significant role in the development or exacerbation of other psychiatric disorders, including depression and substance abuse, and are often associated with a variety of medical illnesses (Starcevic, 2005).

Although the onset of anxiety disorders can occur at any age, they are most likely to begin in childhood or early adulthood, and frequently take a chronic course (Vasey & Dadds, 2001). Much of the research conducted on anxiety disorders has focused on younger populations. There is relatively little available information about the onset of anxiety, its etiology, and the nature of its course for the elderly, in general, and for older women in particular. This paper provides an overview of the diagnostic criteria for the major anxiety disorders, excluding posttraumatic stress disorder (PTSD). With a special emphasis on women and aging, information regarding anxiety disorders is provided on prevalence, etiology, assessment, treatment, and the need for additional research.

ANXIETY DISORDERS:
DESCRIPTION AND DIAGNOSIS

According to the Diagnostic and Statistical Manual of Mental Disorders, Text Revision (DSM-IV-TR; American Psychiatric Association, 2000), anxiety disorders are classified into several major subtypes. Five of these subtypes are described as follows.

1. Panic Disorder refers to a syndrome of repeated and unexpected panic or anxiety attacks, where an individual experiences discrete episodes of intense fear, trembling, shortness of breath, sweating, dizziness and/or a fear of going crazy. Panic disorder can occur alone, or in conjunction with agoraphobia, which is best summarized as a fear of being in certain situations, such as traveling alone, going outside of the house or being in crowds. Often travel outside the house is limited and/or certain situations are completely avoided. It is rare that agoraphobia will occur without panic disorder.

2. The main features of a Specific Phobia include an excessive and irrational fear of a specific situation, or the anticipation of exposure to such. Fear may be related to a strong concern about potential harm, losing control, or disgust. Typically, when exposed to a phobic situation, individuals will immediately experience anxiety, and the degree of fear is related to the proximity of the trigger as well as avenues of possible escape. The DSM-IV-TR distinguishes among common subtypes of specific phobias, which include animal type, natural environment type (e.g., storms, heights), blood-injection-injury type, and situational type (e.g., bridges, flying).

3. Social Phobia is defined as a significant and ongoing unreasonable fear that is related to one's social interaction or performance (or anticipation of such) in social situations. Typically, an individual fears that when in new or unfamiliar situations, he or she will act in a manner that will be judged negatively by others, resulting in humiliation. People with social phobia believe others will view them as weak, stupid or inept in the context of their interactions. Consequently, people with social phobia will often avoid these fearful situations, or endure them only with great discomfort.

4. Obsessive Compulsive Disorder (OCD) refers to a condition that involves either recurrent obsessions and/or compulsions that are time consuming and cause significant impairment in a person's daily functioning. Obsessions are defined as unwanted recurrent thoughts, ideas or impulses that are intrusive and uncontrollable, and which cause considerable distress. The content of obsessions can vary, with the most common themes including thoughts of contamination, repeated doubts, a need to arrange things in a particular way, and unpleasant aggressive or sexual thoughts.

Compulsions are defined as repetitive actions, which could be overt behaviors (e.g., hand washing, checking, or hoarding) or covert ones (e.g., counting), whose purpose is to reduce or neutralize the anxiety generated by the person's obsessive preoccupations.

5. Generalized Anxiety Disorder (GAD) is characterized by excessive worry and apprehension about a number of areas in one's life. Typically, individuals with GAD have difficulty controlling their anxiety, and as a result, may experience sleep difficulty, irritability, difficulty with concentration, and muscle tension. People with GAD often worry about issues that are trivial, or about real issues that are grossly blown of out proportion. Because of the excessive nature of their worrying, it is not uncommon for individuals with GAD to have difficulty functioning across a wide range of social and vocational situations.

PREVALENCE RATES FOR ANXIETY DISORDERS

The lifetime prevalence rate of panic disorder is between 1.7% and 3.5% in community samples. Myers et al. (cited in Fisher, 2001) noted that among the elderly, including those 65 years and older, the six-month prevalence rate for panic disorder was 2% for females and 0% for males. The six-month prevalence rate for agoraphobia was 3.0% for females and 1.6% for males. Women with panic disorder without agoraphobia outnumber men almost 2:1, and women with panic disorder with agoraphobia outnumber men about 3:1.

Specific phobias are relatively common in the general population. In fact, prevalence rates in community samples range from 4% to 8%. Lifetime prevalence rates range from 7.2% to 12.5% (American Psychiatric Association, 2000). Myers et al. (cited in Fisher, 2001) found the six-month prevalence rate to be 7.0% for females and 3.3% for males, 65 years and older. Women tend to outnumber men approximately 2:1 with regard to specific phobias. This ratio changes depending on the type of specific phobia, with women accounting for 75% to 90% of persons with animal, natural environment and situation type phobias, and 50% to 70% of those with blood-injection type phobia.

The lifetime prevalence rate for social phobia ranges from 3% to 13%, according to epidemiological and community samples (American Psychiatric Association, 2000). Approximately one third of individuals with social phobia are fearful of public speaking. Another one third of persons are fearful of at least one other social situation, such as talking to strangers. The remaining one third of individuals are fearful of multiple social situations. Social phobia tends to appear more frequently in women in community samples. The prevalence rate is almost the same for women as for men in clinical samples (Starcevic, 2005).

With regard to OCD, the lifetime prevalence rate ranges from 1.5% to 2.5% in community samples (Starcevic, 2005; Steketee & Barlow, 2004). A one-year prevalence rate is estimated at 0.5% to 2.1% for the adult population, with OCD being approximately equally divided between men and women (American Psychiatric Association, 2000). OCD is more commonly found in male children and adolescents than in females. Within the elderly population, Myers et al. (cited in Fisher, 2001), found that 1.0% of females and 1.3% of males 65 years and older experienced OCD.

Epidemiology rates concerning GAD have been inconsistent, largely as a result of changing methodologies employed in studies, as well as changing criteria for GAD over time (Roemer, Orsillo, & Barlow, 2004). However, it is generally accepted that the one-year prevalence rate for GAD is approximately 3%, with a lifetime prevalence rate of about 5% (American Psychiatric Association, 2000; Roemer et al., 2004). About two thirds of all GAD sufferers tend to be women, and it is one of the most frequently occurring disorders found in all age groups, including the elderly (Starcevic, 2005). Blazer, George and Hughes (cited in Scogin, 1998) noted in their study that almost half of the elderly participants age 65 and older who had GAD suffered from symptoms for less than five years. This suggests that late onset GAD is more prevalent than originally thought. GAD is often associated with other medical and psychological conditions, and prevalence rates in primary care settings are high (Roemer et al., 2004).

TYPICAL COURSE OF ANXIETY DISORDERS

The onset of panic disorder can occur at any age, although it is not as common in children and in the elderly. Onset usually begins either in the 15-24 year-old group or in the 45-54 year-old group (Starcevic, 2005). Panic disorder is a chronic condition for the majority of patients, with only 30% to 35% of patients experiencing a nearly complete recovery. In addition, approximately 50% of patients have a chronic, but fluctuating course, and 15% to 20% have a chronic course without fluctuation. A number of factors are predictive of the course of panic disorder, particularly involving a poor outcome. They include being unpartnered, early onset of panic disorder, longer period of time before seeking treatment, high severity of symptoms, co-occurrence of a personality disorder and/or a depressive disorder, and poor response to initial treatment (Starcevic, 2005).

Although the onset for specific phobias tends to begin in childhood or adolescence, it can vary depending on the type of phobia. For instance, situational phobias often begin in childhood and then reoccur in the early to the mid-20s. The onset of specific phobias related to the natural environment can vary greatly, occurring in either childhood or adulthood. In contrast, specific phobias related to the animal type and blood-injection-injury type usually begin in childhood (Antony & Barlow, 2002; Starcevic, 2005).

The course of specific phobias can vary greatly, ranging from remission to ongoing chronicity. At this time, it is not known whether one type of specific phobia is more likely to remit than another. However, what triggers the onset and the longevity of the phobic/avoidance response most likely play crucial roles in the course of the specific phobia. Phobias that begin in childhood and continue into adulthood have only a 20% chance of remission (Starcevic, 2005). Specific phobias often occur with other anxiety disorders, depression or substance abuse. Comorbidity rates with specific phobias range from 50% to 80% of community samples. Unfortunately, unless an individual is experiencing major distress due to the presence of a specific phobia, it is unlikely that he or she will seek necessary treatment (American Psychiatric Association, 2000).

The average age of onset for social phobia is between 15 and 16 years. It usually occurs slowly, often emerging from childhood shyness. The course of the disorder is typically chronic, with few fluctuations (American Psychiatric Association, 2000). There have been several variables associated with a poor prognosis for social phobia and they include early onset, severity of symptoms, co-morbidity with other psychiatric disorders, presence of a mood disorder, health problems, and lower educational achievement (Starcevic, 2005). Social phobia frequently co-occurs with other psychiatric disorders such as depression, other anxiety disorders, alcohol abuse and personality disorders (Rubin & Burgess, 2001).

OCD usually begins in early adulthood, with a mean age of onset between 21 and 22 years of age. Onset for males is earlier, often occurring between the ages of six and 15. For females, the onset is usually later between the ages of 20 and 29 (American Psychiatric Association, 2000). Almost 80% of individuals with OCD report an onset after the age of 14. Typically, onset of OCD is a slow and gradual process. For most individuals, the course of OCD is a chronic condition, with fluctuating symptoms (American Psychiatric Association, 2000). Fewer than 20% of all patients with OCD report a complete recovery from this disorder

(Starcevic, 2005). It is estimated that more than half of all OCD patients also suffer from another type of anxiety disorder and/or depression (Steketee & Barlow, 2004). Predictors for a poor prognosis for those with OCD include: early onset, being single, greater severity and longer duration of symptoms, presence of delusions, magical thinking, presence of a personality disorder, presence of bipolar and/or eating disorder, and impaired social functioning.

More than half of all individuals who suffer from GAD report an onset beginning in childhood or adolescence. The most common age range for onset of this disorder is between 15 and 25 years. Onset is usually gradual, and GAD tends to be a chronic condition whose symptoms fluctuate over time. Those symptoms generally intensify during times when a person's external life circumstances become stressful (American Psychiatric Association, 2000; Starcevic, 2005). For approximately 67% of persons with GAD, there is a co-occurring mental disorder, most typically depressive disorder, other anxiety disorders, or substance abuse (Roemer, Orsillo, & Barlow, 2004).

ETIOLOGY OF ANXIETY DISORDERS

The etiology of anxiety disorders is not fully understood. However, major theories have been postulated in an attempt to explain the origins of anxiety. For the most part, proposed models for anxiety disorders typically include biological and psychological constructs. A brief review of some of the relevant theories and variables relevant to the development of anxiety is presented below.

Psychoanalytic Theory. According to psychoanalytic thought, anxiety is produced as a result of unconscious conflicts and issues. It is postulated that there is a conflict between one's sexual or aggressive urges and the defenses an individual employs to deal with these urges (Brill, 1995). The purpose of psychoanalytic therapy is to help an individual gain insight into his or her unconscious conflicts, thereby resolving the conflict and freeing the person from the anxieties. Although this model was very popular during the previous century, it has not held up well to scientific scrutiny and is now considered controversial (Starcevic, 2005).

Behavioral Theory. This psychological model posits that feelings of anxiety result from learning, via classical and instrumental conditioning. For example, as a result of an aversive experience, an individual will learn to associate a neutral stimulus with feelings of danger or vulnerability. As a consequence of this negative emotional association, even in subsequent situations that are not aversive, the neutral stimulus alone will be enough to elicit an anxiety response. This anxiety response can become more firmly entrenched if the person then avoids the formerly neutral stimulus. This process of avoidance limits the exposure to the neutral stimulus and makes it unlikely that the individual will be able to habituate or relearn that the neutral stimulus is not threatening (Rapee & Barlow, 2004). Sometimes criticized as being overly simplistic, behavioral therapy is one of the most effective treatments for anxiety disorders (Starcevic, 2005).

Cognitive Theory. Cognitive models of anxiety disorders focus on an individual's faulty and distorted appraisal of potential danger. For example, anxious individuals were more likely than normal control subjects to interpret ambiguous situations or environmental stimuli as potentially threatening, which they believe could result in potential harm or even death (Rapee & Barlow, 2004). Although cognitive models have become increasingly popular as a treatment approach, they have not been rigorously tested, and it is not clear whether cognitive-oriented treatment is as effective as behavior therapies (Starcevic, 2005).

Genetic and Familial Factors. There is an increasing amount of evidence that hereditary factors play a significant role in the development of anxiety disorders. Barlow (2004) summarized family studies and indicated that patients with panic disorder and agoraphobia were much more likely to have relatives with the disorder than relatives of patients who did not have this disorder. Prevalence rates for family members of the former group ranged from 7.9% to 41%. The prevalence rate for the control group was never above 8%. High concordance rates for family members of patients with GAD, OCD, social and specific phobias have been reported as well (American Psychiatric Association, 2000; Rapee & Barlow, 2004). While twin studies have revealed a genetic contribution to anxiety, the results for some family and twin studies may have been confounded by shared environmental experiences (Starcevic, 2005).

Biological Factors. Several neurotransmitter systems have been identified as possibly being associated with the development of anxiety disorders. They include: norepinephrine, serotonin, and gamma-aminobutyric acid (GABA). Studies of neurotransmitter system abnormalities have typically resulted from interest in the effects certain medications (e.g., buspirone, benzodiazepines) may have on these systems. Results of these studies tend to be inconclusive as specific anxiety disorders have not been associated with specific neurotransmitter abnormalities. When abnormalities are observed, it is unclear if they occurred prior to, or as a result of an anxiety disorder.

Sociocultural Factors. While the evidence is clear that women are more likely to suffer from an anxiety disorder than men, the reasons for these research findings are not clear. Possible explanations to account for these differences have included differences in parenting styles and gender roles, the tendency for females toward greater negative affectivity, and the interaction of physiology and behavior on the development of anxiety disorders (Craske, 2003; Hazlett-Stevens, 2005). Another possible link between the development of anxiety disorders and sociocultural factors is the role of social reinforcement. Social reinforcement influences gender roles beginning in childhood. For example, parents typically reinforce male children to be assertive, active and independent. However, female children are frequently encouraged to be cautious and less independent, and so their behavior is typically more controlled. As a result, boys are exposed to a broader range of experiences and tend to be more self-reliant. Males are also thought to develop more effective coping skills that serve to reduce the amount of negative reactivity they experience throughout their lifetime when exposed to stressful situations (Craske, 2003; Hazlett-Stevens, 2005).

Another sociocultural factor implicated in the vulnerability to anxiety in females is that women are prone to display higher levels of negative affectivity. This tendency begins in early childhood and sex differences become more pronounced as age increases. Females tend to exhibit increased levels of negative affectivity as they get older whereas males are likely to remain somewhat constant with regard to this trait. The higher levels of negative affectivity that women experience are associated with a tendency to ruminate about the problems they encounter throughout their lives. This combination of negative affectivity and the tendency to ruminate predisposes women to be more likely to recognize perceived threats, to fear specific objects or situations, and to respond more emotionally to negative situations than do men. Such distress may interfere with one's ability to effectively cope, and lead to increased levels of anxiety (Craske, 2003; Hazlett-Stevens, 2005).

Finally, studies concerning anxiety and its relationship to physiology and behavior suggest that there are differences between male and female responses to acute stress (Craske, 2003). For example, both males and females experience "fight or flight" responses when in stressful situations. One manifestation of this response is an increase in activity in the adrenal medullary and hypothalamic-pituitary systems. However, only in the females is there a dampening effect of this response, which is thought to be caused by oxytocin and endogenous opiates. In behavioral terms, what results is that women show a blunted response to "fight or flight," which may have evolutionary implications. For instance, by not fighting or fleeing, women can focus their energies on caring for their young and befriending others. This type of a response lends itself to the formation of social groups for the purpose of security and preservation. A possible negative consequence of the development of this "tend and befriend" response may be that it causes women to internalize negative emotions instead of expressing them. These tendencies can lead women to ruminate about stressful situations and/or act in ways that are concil-iatory in order to keep the peace as a means of coping with stressful events. In contrast, males who experience a stronger "fight or flight" re-sponse are more likely to act in ways that expose them to potential con-flict and trauma. This exposure provides them with more opportunities to master stressful events in ways that foster independence and self-con-fidence. These sociocultural differences may make males feel more in control of their circumstances. As a result, males appear to be less prone to experience prolonged feelings of anxiety (Craske, 2003; Hazlett-Stevens, 2005).

Adult Developmental Milestones, Anxiety, and Co-Morbidity. Al-though most anxiety disorders begin in childhood or early adulthood, there is growing recognition that some anxiety disorders begin in later life. Despite the fact that the etiology of late onset anxiety is not well-understood (Zarit & Zarit, 1998), it is important to identify possi-ble triggers as well as life experiences often associated with the late on-set of anxiety.

For the most part, anxiety in later life has been associated with vari-ous psychiatric and medical disorders (Hidalgo & Davidson, 2001). In addition, psychosocial issues, such as loss of family members and friends, and retirement from gainful employment are linked to anxiety disorders in the elderly (Wartenberg & Nirenberg, 1995). In an effort to better understand the onset of anxiety disorders in the elderly, a brief re-view of the significant factors that can trigger the development of an anxiety disorder late in life, or exacerbate a preexisting anxiety disorder will be presented.

Medical Factors. It would appear that medical illnesses play a unique and complex role in the development of anxiety disorders in the elderly. Wells, Golding, and Burnam (cited in Cassem, 1990) found that indi-viduals with one or more medical conditions had a six-month preva-lence rate of 24.7%, and a lifetime prevalence rate of 42.2% of having a psychiatric disorder. The most common psychiatric disorder associated with medical illness was substance abuse, followed by anxiety and affective disorders. Despite the fact that medical illnesses can complicate the course of an anxiety disorder as well as other psychiatric conditions, medical conditions may be overlooked as a concurrent illness. Hidalgo and Davidson (2001) and Raj and Sheehan (cited in Zarit & Zarit, 1998) present lists of medical disorders often associated with anxiety disorders in the elderly. These illnesses include osteoporosis, asthma, diabetes, thyroid problems, allergies, hip, joint and back difficulties, cardiac disease, chronic obstructive pulmonary disease (COPD), neurological diseases and hypertension. An in-depth look at several commonly occurring medical problems and their relationship to anxiety in the elderly will be examined.

Dementia (a brain disorder that impairs memory and at least one additional area of cognitive functioning) is known to occur more frequently in the elderly, with a slightly higher prevalence rate for females than for males (American Psychiatric Association, 2000). Because dementia affects an individual's cognitive functioning in different ways, impairment in judgment, language, spatial skills, and memory will occur in varying combinations. Such impairment has implications for changes in behavioral and emotional functioning which may cause an individual to experience levels of anxiety capable of triggering an anxiety disorder (Fromholt & Bruhn, 1998). As a result, a person's daily routines, whether they include social, vocational or leisure time activities, are often compromised. Tragically, deficits due to dementia can cause a person's world to appear distorted, challenging and threatening. Depending on how intact an individual's level of awareness is regarding the changes in their cognitive functioning, they can experience significant and sometimes overwhelming stress, worry and anxiety.

Another aspect of aging is the various changes the eye undergoes that can negatively affect an individual's vision. These changes can have a negative impact on emotional well-being. For instance, changes in the eye's lens, retina, and vitreous humor can adversely impact a person's visual acuity in terms of clarity, color discrimination, and ability to see objects at close distance. Age-related changes can also affect one's sensitivity to light, visual acuity in areas of poor illumination, and stereoscopic visions (Whitbourne, 1998). All of these changes can place significant limitations on an individual's ability to participate in a variety of life activities (e.g., reading, driving). As a result of these limitations and the problems they create, individuals afflicted often experience increased levels of anxiety. There are also a number of specific eye diseases that frequently occur in the elderly which can adversely impact a person's vision. These diseases include: cataracts, macular degeneration, glaucoma, and diabetic retinopathy. For many individuals, visual impairment is frequently treatable through surgery, correction with prescription glasses, and/or by providing increased lighting. However, for some individuals, intervention is not an option, or if undertaken, may prove ineffective.

The psychological implications of impaired vision among the elderly can have far reaching consequences. For instance, problems with depth perception and visual acuity at night, could put an individual at risk for falls, which could lead to serious injury. Poor vision may impair one's ability to live independently, and an individual's cooking, bill paying, shopping, and traveling abilities could therefore be significantly limited. Impairment in leisure time activities such as gardening, painting, and sewing may be another consequence of poor vision (Whitbourne, 1998). Vocational limitations may also result from poor vision, as a person's ability to read, write, or use a computer, and perhaps most significantly the ability to drive, could be negatively impaired. Given the restrictions imposed by poor vision on many activities, it is not surprising that many people respond with feelings of stress, worry, and anxiety.

Another sensory loss experienced by the elderly is presbycusis or age-related hearing loss. Although there are several subtypes of hearing loss, the most common form of this disorder is a reduction in sensitivity to high frequency tones. For many individuals, hearing loss can begin as early as 40 years of age, with the greatest percentage of persons experiencing hearing loss between the ages of 70 and 80. Typically, hearing loss is more common in men than in women (Whitbourne, 1998).

The psychological implications for hearing loss can be significant. Relationships with others can be altered and/or strained as a result. Verbal exchanges can be difficult, with significant portions of conversations being misinterpreted and/or completely ignored by a hearing impaired individual. Also, safety issues are a matter of concern for individuals with hearing loss, as they may not be able to detect a knock on the door, to discern the sirens of passing fire trucks or ambulances, or to appreciate the content of important broadcasts over loudspeakers or television (Whitbourne, 1998). There is clear evidence that social isolation resulting from hearing impairment can cause people to feel lonely, sad, and isolated and that those feelings can lead to significant episodes of emotional distress, including feelings of anxiety.

Another age-related change in sensory function is in the vestibular system, which can result in dizziness and vertigo in older individuals. In addition to psychiatric and medical illnesses, dizziness can be caused or exacerbated by illicit drugs, alcohol, and prescription medications (Whitbourne, 1998). There are often significant emotional implications for those individuals who suffer from balance problems. Many of those emotional issues are related to safety. More specifically, the possibility of falls and subsequent injury are of great concern for this group of individuals. In addition, social relationships can be negatively affected by balance problems. Because balance problems make the navigation of one's environment more challenging and potentially dangerous, some individuals with vestibular problems may limit contact with others by withdrawing into the safety of their own homes. For those who maintain contact, the social presentation of individuals with balance difficulties may be compromised, as they may appear stooped or hunched over. This may give the impression that a person is confused or intoxicated. As a consequence, these types of social interactions may lead to potentially embarrassing situations, which in turn can cause individuals to withdraw socially and to experience feelings of loneliness, increased levels of anxiety and depression (Whitbourne, 1998).

According to Busby-Whitehead (1995), approximately 15%-20% of community dwelling individuals over the age of 65 are affected by urinary incontinence. Prevalence rates for urinary incontinence are higher for patients in acute care facilities and nursing homes. Females are at greater risk than males for developing this medical problem. Fecal incontinence is not an unusual occurrence in the elderly as well, although it affects a minority of individuals (Norton, 1995). Despite the fact that there are a number of available treatments for incontinence, there are individuals who do not respond favorably to these interventions. The psychological implications for these individuals can be significant. Incontinence can interfere with an individual's daily routines, as social events are often avoided and/or endured with great distress, for fear of embarrassment. Many elderly individuals associate incontinence with dementia, and as a result, fear possible institutionalization. Because of an individual's excretory problems, diet might be adversely affected in an effort to limit potentially embarrassing situations. Nutritionally healthy food may be neglected, which could contribute to physical decline and emotional distress. Understandably, anxiety is often a result of incontinence (Whitbourne, 1998).

Psychosocial Factors. By virtue of living a long life, elderly individuals are exposed to varying degrees of loss across a life span. Such losses have the potential to exert a greater impact on an individual's emotional functioning. Nakra (1990) identified potential risk factors for psychiatric illness in the elderly, which can be framed as a form of loss. These include unemployment, diminished income, changes in living arrangements, and loss of friends and family. These events are most commonly associated with the death of others and/or relocation.

Unemployment and diminished income often occur concurrently within the elderly population. Loss of work can result from retirement, disability, or change in domicile. For many individuals, cessation of work results in financial hardship and emotional stress. The emotional impact of diminished income can adversely affect self-esteem as an individual may no longer be able to provide for his/her family as before. An unemployed elderly person may no longer be able to provide the financial assistance to significant others on birthdays or holidays, with home repairs, or with college tuition for grandchildren. Lifestyle changes may be required if an individual is no longer earning the same wages that were required to pay for rent/mortgage, dining out, medicine, and health insurance. Finally, relationships with family members and friends may be strained because of decreased contact with others, as there may not be the necessary funds available to travel to see loved ones.

Changes in living arrangements can have a significant impact on a person's emotional well-being. In an AARP study, 86% of individuals interviewed indicated that their preference was to remain in their own homes (cited in Glassman, 1995). By doing so, individuals remain connected to their community and thereby retain a sense of identity and self-esteem. A person's home is a center for family and social events. It can be a symbol of one's independence and mastery over one's life. Relocation, either forced or voluntary, can result in feelings of loss, incompetence, and decreased self-esteem. As a consequence, psychological disorders, including anxiety disorders, may result. Research has demonstrated that people are particularly vulnerable when relocated to a nursing home facility, where prevalence rates of psychiatric illness are high (Zarit & Zarit, 1998).

In terms of gender differences, women are thought to be less at risk for experiencing the impact of events related to psychosocial losses than men because they typically have larger social support networks, have more frequent contact with friends and family, including children, and are more likely to be living with another person(s) than are men. However, given that women tend to live longer than men, they also have more opportunities to experience those psychosocial losses and their associated consequences. For example, although widowhood is a significant emotional trauma for both sexes, because women tend to outlive men they are at higher risk for experiencing this event.

In general, the elderly experience multiple types of losses (physical, social and situational), and the likelihood of sustaining multiple losses increases the longer they survive the aging process. The types of losses associated with old age have also been linked with a diminished ability to access much-needed social support networks when in time of crisis and need (Rakowski, Pearlman, & Murphy, 1995). In sum, the longer people live and the more losses they experience, the more trauma and distress they are exposed to without the supports they need to cope with those losses. The formation of psychiatric disorders, including anxiety disorder, is often the consequence of such losses.

ASSESSMENT AND TREATMENT

There is relatively little available treatment research regarding the elderly and anxiety disorders. Research that does exist suggests that most geriatric individuals do not seek treatment for anxiety disorders. For the minority of individuals who do seek treatment, it is often through their primary care physician, who frequently prescribes medication. Currently, treatment procedures for anxiety disorders are typically the same for all age groups. Some of the more common treatment techniques will be presented below and can be used as models of possible treatment for the elderly.

Panic Disorder. When a panic disorder is suspected, a comprehensive evaluation should be undertaken, such as routine medical studies, including a laboratory workup and possibly a neurological examination. In addition, psychological interviews, including those based on DSM-IV-TR criteria and various self-report scales/measures, such as the Panic Disorder Severity Scale (PDSS) and the Panic and Agoraphobia Scale, may be used by trained health professionals (Starcevic, 2005; White & Barlow, 2004).

Treatment for panic disorder usually consists of pharmacological and/or psychosocial interventions (Starcevic, 2005; White & Barlow, 2004). Pharmacological intervention is usually applied when an individual is experiencing at least moderate discomfort. Three groups of medications are frequently used in the treatment of panic disorder: Tricyclic Antidepressants (TCAs), Selective Serotonin Reuptake Inhibitors (SSRIs), and benzodiazepines (Roy-Byrne & Cowley, 1998;

White & Barlow, 2004). These medications may be used alone or in combination with each other. Pharmacological treatment typically continues for 6-12 months after an individual goes into remission.

Psychosocial treatment models usually consist of cognitive-behavioral therapy (CBT), psychodynamic psychotherapy, and other psychotherapeutic techniques, such as exposure therapy and relaxation techniques. CBT tends to focus on identifying an individual's faulty thought processes (e.g., irrational and catastrophic beliefs about a particular situation) and replacing those beliefs with more rational ones. Behavioral treatment may include gradual exposure to anxiety-provoking situations until the anxiety dissipates and habituation occurs (Starcevic, 2005). Psychodynamic approaches focus on gaining insight about unconscious conflicts (e.g., fear of abandonment) and their origins. The goal is to resolve the unconscious conflicts which can then free a person from experiencing unnecessary anxiety. Finally, relaxation techniques, including deep breathing exercises, can be used to contain feelings of panic. It is important to note that many individuals with panic disorder seek professional help, although they are often found in medical clinics or emergency rooms of hospitals because of the somatic symptoms they experience. Unfortunately, within such treatment settings, the diagnosis of an anxiety disorder may be overlooked, or the immediate episode is treated and the patient is released (Starcevic, 2005). If they are fortunate they may be advised to seek mental health care.

Specific Phobia. The assessment of a phobia typically consists of a diagnostic interview conducted by a trained health-care provider. DSM-IV-TR criteria are used to make the diagnosis. Assessment instruments, such as the Fear Questionnaire (FQ), can be used to determine the presence of any type of phobia (cited in Fischer & Corcoran, 1994).

It is commonly accepted that the most successful treatment for phobia consists of some variation of behaviorally oriented exposure therapy (Antony & Barlow, 2004). This treatment technique exposes an individual to the feared phobic stimulus, thus allowing the individual to experience that nothing aversive actually occurs. In the process a person becomes habituated to the feared stimulus and as a consequence no longer ruminates about, or avoids the previously feared stimulus. Although post-treatment follow-up studies have been mixed, it is believed that most people do not relapse after successful treatment (Antony & Barlow, 2004).

Social Phobia. As for other anxiety disorders, the diagnosis of social phobia is made by a trained professional, using DSM-IV-TR criteria.

Assessment instruments may be employed as well, and can include the Liebowitz Social Anxiety Scale (LSAS) and the Brief Social Phobia Scale (cited in Hofmann & Barlow, 2004).

CBT is often employed in the treatment of social phobia. CBT focuses on uncovering the cognitive distortions or faulty assumptions individuals internalize regarding underlying assumptions and the social world. In the case of social anxiety, people view themselves as generally incompetent and believe that others are constantly evaluating them negatively. These two factors interact in ways that make the person perceive having social contact with others as threatening. The goal of treatment is to examine the evidence in their lives and challenge the distorted underlying ideas. As a result patients construct a more positive and realistic appraisal of themselves and their interactions with other people.

Cognitive reconstruction is usually paired with exposure-based interventions. The exposure is done gradually, and is based upon a patient's hierarchy of least to most anxiety-provoking social situations. This gradual exposure to the feared social situations facilitates the patient's ability to face those fears, and garner evidence that challenges the cognitive distortions. The intended result of treatment is that the patient begins to develop a comfort level in social situations that were previously viewed as threatening.

It is not uncommon in clinical practice to combine various aspects of CBT with pharmacological intervention. However, it is not known how these treatments should be optimally combined (Starcevic, 2005). Finally, it is important to note that Regier et al. (cited in Starcevic, 2005) found that 73%-87% of persons suffering from social phobia do not seek treatment. Of those individuals who do participate in treatment, intervention usually commences about 10 or more years after the onset of social phobia.

Obsessive-Compulsive Disorder. OCD is diagnosed in a manner similar to the other anxiety disorders. Frequently an assessment instrument such as the Yale-Brown Obsessive Scale (YBOCS) (cited in Steketee & Barlow 2004) is used in making the diagnosis.

Treatment for OCD usually consists of pharmacological and/or psychological interventions. Psychological interventions usually consist of exposure and response prevention (behavioral therapy) and/or cognitive behavior therapy (CBT) (Franklin & Foa, 1998; Steketee & Barlow, 2004). As in the treatment of social phobia, CBT focuses on identifying cognitive distortions. In the case of OCD these irrational ideas are related to core beliefs that perpetuate obsessive ruminations and compulsive behaviors.

Treatment strategies for OCD usually involve the technique of exposure and response prevention. The initial stage of treatment involves prolonged exposure to the feared stimulus situation, followed by response prevention (e.g., no ritualistic behavior). Exposure is gradual and involves the patient constructing a hierarchy of least to most feared situations. These can include real as well as imagined situations. In general, patients work through their hierarchy by confronting the feared situations and at the same time being willing to abstain from engaging in the compulsive rituals they had previously employed to make themselves feel safe. This combination of exposure and response prevention allows them to habituate and to learn, experientially, that nothing bad will happen to them as a result. Successful treatment leads to an improved sense of self-control (Franklin & Foa, 1998; Steketee & Barlow, 2004).

Despite available treatments for OCD, it is rare that a complete remission will occur. Rather, the often stated goal of contemporary treatment is a lessening of the person's symptoms, which leads to improvement in a person's day-to-day living. Often patients resist seeking treatment for OCD. Starcevic (2005) cited a study that found that patients with OCD often waited an average of 7.5 years before seeking treatment.

Generalized Anxiety Disorder. DSM-IV-TR criteria are used to make a diagnosis of GAD. A trained health-care provider conducts the diagnostic interview using common assessment instruments, such as the Penn State Worry Questionnaire (Starcevic, 2005). Because GAD frequently co-occurs with physical illness and/or drug conditions, a complete medical examination, including laboratory study, is recommended.

Treatment for GAD typically consists of psychological and/or pharmacological interventions. The psychological treatment for GAD usually takes the form of cognitive, behavioral, or supportive therapy (Roemer et al, 2004; Starcevic, 2005). Cognitive therapy for GAD is similar in technique to that used for other anxiety disorders. It involves identifying the underlying faulty belief system, and replacing it with more rational thought processes. Psycho-educational interventions are frequently employed as a means of teaching an individual about fear and its physiological, behavioral, and emotional consequences. This intervention helps empower the patient to understand the nature of the disorder and teaches them the skills to actively cope with symptoms. Behavioral techniques often include imaginal and in vivo exposure to stressful situations, along with instruction in relaxation exercises and other coping skills to manage the physical sensations, thoughts, and feelings associated with GAD.

Pharmacological treatment usually consists of Venlafaxine (Effexor) or an SSRI. Other medications that may be used in treatment of GAD include: benzodiazepines, buspirone, hydroxyzine, and beta blockers (Roemer et al., 2004; Starcevic, 2005).

WOMEN, AGING, AND ANXIETY

The epidemiological data clearly indicate that older women are more likely to develop anxiety disorders than older men. Despite the fact that relatively little is known about the etiology of anxiety disorders in older women, preliminary evidence indicates that medical, psychosocial, and substance usage factors play a significant role.

One of the areas in which the gerontology literature presents clear findings is establishing a link between medical problems and the development of anxiety disorders in elderly women. For example, if an elderly person has one or more medical problems, there is a significantly higher risk of developing a psychiatric disorder (Cassem, 1990). This finding is particularly significant, as women are at greater risk than men for suffering from a variety of medical conditions. Urinary incontinence is a medical problem that is more often found in older women. The psychological implications of suffering with incontinence are significant. Avoidance of social events due to the anticipatory fear of embarrassment generally has a negative impact on the quality of life for elderly females who experience episodes of urinary incontinence. Ambivalence and anticipatory anxiety regarding social relationships can lead to the development of anxiety disorder.

Elderly women also commonly experience medical problems related to sensory deficits, such as impaired hearing, vision, and balance. These deficits raise concerns related to compromised ability to function regarding living independently, working, traveling, socializing, and attending to their physical health and safety (Whitbourne, 1998). Restrictions in lifestyle and worries that women have regarding their personal safety related to sensory deficits have been associated with onset of anxiety.

In the final analysis, simply by the fact that women live longer than men, women are more at risk for developing one or more of the many illnesses often associated with aging, including Parkinson's Disease,

Chronic Obstructive Pulmonary Disease (COPD), thyroid problems, arthritis, and cardiac disease (Zarit & Zarit, 1998). These and other medical problems create serious restrictions in lifestyle and significant worries regarding the quality of their relationships with others as well as their sense of their own mortality. These restrictions, worries and fears contribute to the development of anxiety disorder or the exacerbation of preexisting anxiety disorders in elderly women.

Another psychosocial factor that is associated with anxiety disorders in elderly women is their living arrangements. Many older women have attempted to remain in their long-standing place of residence after experiencing milestone events such as retirement, physical illness, or loss of a spouse. Unfortunately, any of these events could result in hardship for elderly women who are attempting to maintain a household. Homes are a source of pleasant memories for many individuals and provide a sense of belonging to a community. It is understandable why older women would be reluctant to give up such a residence, as well as respond to this dilemma with anxiety (Glassman, 1995). In contrast, some elderly women desire a change in residence, but are unable to relocate, possibly as a result of financial limitations. One consequence may be to continue to live in a crime-ridden area, which is very stressful. An equally difficult situation may include a move to a nursing home, where psychiatric illness rates are high (Zarit & Zarit, 1998).

One final psychosocial factor to consider regarding older women and anxiety disorders is their social support network. Typically, older females have stronger social support systems than elderly men, who tend to be socially isolated. Often, elderly women have more friends than elderly men; in addition, they have an increased likelihood of living with a close friend or family member. As a result, however, the women run the risk of experiencing more losses than elderly men. As they suffer these types of losses, they may also experience a loss of important roles. As a consequence, their sense of purpose and identity may be challenged in ways that lead to the development of anxiety. Finally, although older males are at higher risk for mortality when losing a spouse, the risk is not insignificant for elderly women (Rakowski et al., 1995).

The use of substances by elderly females is an important factor in the development of an anxiety disorder. Although older women are not as likely as older men to abuse alcohol or illegal substances, they are at risk for abusing prescription medications, which are frequently prescribed for treatment of sleep problems, pain, or another medical condition. Abuse or multiple use of medications can lead to disruption in cognitive and emotional functioning (Wartenberg & Nirenberg, 1995).

FUTURE DIRECTIONS

Anxiety is one of the most commonly occurring psychiatric disorders. It occurs more frequently in females than in males and is often associated with difficulty in social, academic, or vocational functioning. For many individuals, the onset of anxiety occurs early in life and takes a chronic course. Anxiety can also be a precursor for the development of depression and other psychiatric disorders later in life. At this time, most of the current research concerning the onset, etiology and treatment for anxiety disorders has focused on younger populations. Relatively little is known about the course of anxiety and its treatment in elderly females or the differences between older women and men. Consequently, more research is needed regarding the prevalence rates, onset and etiology of anxiety disorders in elderly women. Developing a greater knowledge base could lead to more public education and more effective treatments. As a result, screening for anxiety disorders could become more effective, and more timely treatment and/or prevention strategies could be implemented when working with older adults.

A related issue is that the literature is not clear if there are significant differences in how anxiety is experienced in younger age groups as compared to the elderly. This could lead to important implications as to whether or not treatment techniques employed with younger individuals need to be modified to enhance their effectiveness when applied to older adults.

More importantly, there is a question as to how best to treat older people who have not sought treatment or have delayed treatment for many years. These individuals have lived for years modifying their lives to avoid or minimize having to experience intense feelings of anxiety. By the time they seek treatment or are pushed into treatment by frustrated family members, many of these individuals are advancing in age. Developing or modifying treatment techniques that can address anxiety disorders that are long-standing or have been tolerated for many years could have significant implications for the emotional well-being of the older population. Attention to educational programs and public awareness campaigns is one avenue to be explored, along with education of health professionals who are less familiar with the early identification of anxiety disorders. These are significant issues that have direct implications for treatment. The psychiatric literature clearly indicates that early intervention often leads to a better treatment prognosis.

REFERENCES

American Psychiatric Association (2000). *Diagnostic and Statistical Manual of Mental Disorders* (4th ed.). Washington, DC: Author.

Antony, M.M., & Barlow, D.H. (2004). Specific Phobias. In D.H. Barlow (Ed.), *Anxiety and its Disorders* (2nd ed.; pp. 380-417). New York: The Guilford Press.

Barlow, D.H. (2004). The Experience of Anxiety: Shadow of Intelligence or Specter of Death? In D.H. Barlow (Ed.), *Anxiety and Its Disorders* (2nd ed.; pp. 1-36). New York: The Guilford Press.

Brill, A.A. (1995). *The Basic Writings of Sigmund Freud*. New York: The Modern Library.

Busby-Whitehead, J. (1995). Urinary Incontinence. In W. Reichel (Ed.), *Care of the Elderly* (4th ed.; pp. 280-286). Baltimore: Williams & Wilkins.

Cassem, E.H. (1990). Depression and Anxiety Secondary to Medical Illness. In R.B. Wesner & G. Winokur (Eds.), *Psychiatric Clinics of North America: Anxiety and Depression as Secondary Phenomena*, 13(4) (pp. 597-612). Philadelphia: Saunders.

Craske, M.G. (2003). *Origins of Phobias and Anxiety Disorders: Why More Women than Men?* Oxford: Elsevier.

Craske, M.G., & Chowdhury, N. (2005). Why Are Women Anxious and Worried More Often Than Men? In H. Hazlett-Stevens (Auth.), *Women Who Worry Too Much* (pp. 1-10). Oakland: New Harbinger.

Fischer, J.F., & Corcoran, K. (1994). *Measures for Clinical Practice: A Sourcebook*, 2 (2nd ed.; pp. 340-341). New York: The Free Press.

Fisher, J.E., Zeiss, A.M., & Carstensen, L.L. (2001). Psychopathology in the Aged. In H.E. Adams & P.B. Sutker (Eds.), *Comprehensive Handbook of Psychopathology* (3rd ed.; pp. 921-951). New York: Plenum Publishers.

Franklin, M.E., & Foa, E.B. (1998). Cognitive-Behavioral Treatments for Obsessive Compulsive Disorder. In P.E. Nathan & J.M. Gorman (Eds.), *A Guide to Treatments that Work* (pp. 339-357). New York: Oxford University Press.

Fromholt, P., & Bruhn, P. (1998). Cognitive Dysfunction and Dementia. In I.H. Nordhus, G.R. VandenBos, S. Berg, & P. Fromholt (Eds.), *Clinical Geropsychology* (pp. 183-188).Washington, DC: American Psychological Association.

Glassman, M.H. (1995). Housing for the Elderly. In W. Reichel (Ed.), *Care of the Elderly* (4th ed.; pp. 514-520). Baltimore: Williams & Wilkins.

Hazlett-Stevens, H. (2005). *Women Who Worry Too Much: How to Stop Worry & Anxiety from Ruining Relationships, Work & Fun*. Oakland: New Harbinger.

Hidalgo, R.B., & Davidson, J.R.T. (2001). Generalized Anxiety Disorder: An Important Clinical Concern. *Medical Clinics of North America*, 85(3), 691-710.

Hofmann, S.G., & Barlow, D.H. (2004). Social Phobia (Social Anxiety Disorder). In D.H. Barlow (Ed.), *Anxiety and Its Disorders* (2nd ed.; pp. 454-476). New York: The Guilford Press.

Hume, A.L., & Owens, N.J. (1995). Drugs and the Elderly. In W. Reichel (Ed.), *Care of the Elderly* (4th ed.; pp. 41-63). Baltimore: Williams & Wilkins.

Nakra, B.R.S. (1990). Mood Disorders. In D. Bienenfeld (Ed.), Verwoerdt's *Clinical Geropsychiatry* (3rd ed.; pp. 107-124). Baltimore: Williams & Wilkins.

Norton, R.A. (1995). Gastrointestinal Disease in the Aged. In W. Reichel (Ed.), *Care of the Elderly* (4th ed.; pp. 198-205). Baltimore: Williams & Wilkins.

Rakowski, W., Pearlman, D.N., & Murphy, J.B. (1995). Successful Aging: Psychosocial Factors and Implications for Primary Care Geriatrics. In W. Reichel (Ed.), *Care of the Elderly* (4th ed.; pp. 463-471). Baltimore: Williams & Wilkins.

Rapee, R.M., & Barlow, D.H. (2001). Generalized Anxiety Disorders, Panic Disorders, and Phobias. In H.E. Adams & P.B. Sutker (Eds.), *Comprehensive Handbook of Psychopathology* (3rd ed.; pp. 131-154). New York: Plenum Publishers.

Roemer, L., Orsillo, S.M., & Barlow, D.H. (2004). Generalized Anxiety Disorder. In D.H. Barlow (Ed.), *Anxiety and Its Disorders* (2nd ed.; pp. 477-515). New York: Guilford Press.

Roy-Byrne, P.P., & Cowley, D.S. (1998). Pharmacological Treatment of Panic, Generalized Anxiety, and Phobic Disorders. In P.E. Nathan & J.M. Gorman (Eds.), *A Guide to Treatments that Work* (pp. 319-338). New York: Oxford University Press.

Rubin, K.H., & Burgess, K.B. (2001). Social Withdrawal and Anxiety. In M.W. Vasey & M.R. Dadds (Eds.), *Developmental Psychopathology of Anxiety* (pp. 407-434). New York: Oxford University Press.

Scogin, F.A. (1998). Anxiety in Old Age. In I.H. Nordhus, G.R. VandenBos, S. Berg, & P. Fromholt (Eds.), *Clinical Geropsychology* (pp. 205-209). Washington, DC: American Psychological Association.

Starcevic, V. (2005). *Anxiety Disorders in Adults: A Clinical Guide.* New York: Oxford University Press.

Steketee, G., & Barlow, D.H. (2004). Obsessive-Compulsive Disorder. In D.H. Barlow (Ed.), *Anxiety and Its Disorders* (2nd ed.; pp. 516-550). New York: The Guilford Press.

Vasey, M.W., & Dadds, M.R. (2001). An Introduction to the Developmental Psychopathology of Anxiety. In M.W. Vasey & M.R. Dadds (Eds.), *Developmental Psychopathology of Anxiety* (pp. 3-26). New York: Oxford University Press.

Wartenberg, A.A., & Nirenberg, T.D. (1995). Alcohol and Other Drug Abuse in Older Patients. In W. Reichel (Ed.), *Care of the Elderly: Clinical Aspects of Aging* (4th ed.; pp. 133-141). Baltimore: Williams & Wilkens.

Wesner, R.B. (1990). Alcohol Use and Abuse Secondary to Anxiety. *Psychiatric Clinics of North America: Anxiety and Depression as Secondary Phenomena, 13,* 699-714.

Whitbourne, S.K. (1998). Physical Changes in the Aging Individual: Clinical Implications. In I.H. Nordhus, G.R. VandenBos, S. Berg, & P. Fromholt (Eds.), *Clinical Geropsychology* (pp. 79-108). Washington DC: American Psychological Association.

White, K.S., & Barlow, D.H. (2004). Panic Disorder and Agoraphobia. In D.H. Barlow (Ed.), *Anxiety and Its Disorders* (2nd ed.; pp. 328-379). New York: The Guilford Press.

Zarit, S.H., & Zarit, J.M. (1998). *Mental Disorders in Older Adults: Fundamentals of Assessment and Treatment.* New York: The Guilford Press.

doi:10.1300/J074v19n01_06

Posttraumatic Stress Disorder and Older Women

Miriam Franco, MSW, PsyD

SUMMARY. This article examines the literature related to the identification and treatment of posttraumatic stress disorder in older women. From this review, several key findings emerge. Consistent in the research literature is the fact that American women are more at risk for PTSD than are men as a result of the high frequency of sexual and domestic physical abuse that women experience. Studies on older women and PTSD indicate that older women are under-diagnosed and are more typically perceived as suffering from depression, anxiety or poor physical health. It was found consistently that older women who present with age-related stressors may not be asked about earlier trauma history or it may not be understood within the context of trauma-related variables. In several research studies, trauma history was often not identified either as a result of current assessment practice or because women from certain age cohorts did not disclose trauma-related data to health professionals. Key researchers emphasize the necessity of clinicians, staff and medical personnel to attend to the historical variables present in trauma histories of older women. Researchers underscore the importance of understanding the impact of early and repeated trauma, especially interpersonal trauma, on the physical health and social functioning of older women–

Address correspondence to: Miriam Franco, Sociology Dept., Immaculata University, Immaculata, PA 19345 (E-mail: mfranco@immaculata.edu).

[Haworth co-indexing entry note]: "Posttraumatic Stress Disorder and Older Women." Franco, Miriam. Co-published simultaneously in *Journal of Women & Aging* (The Haworth Press, Inc.) Vol. 19, No. 1/2, 2007, pp. 103-117; and: *Mental Health Issues of Older Women: A Comprehensive Review for Health Care Professionals* (ed: Victor J. Malatesta) The Haworth Press, Inc., 2007, pp. 103-117. Single or multiple copies of this article are available for a fee from The Haworth Document Delivery Service [1-800-HAWORTH, 9:00 a.m. - 5:00 p.m. (EST). E-mail address: docdelivery@haworthpress.com].

even though a significant amount of time may have elapsed since exposure. These findings indicate that further study of PTSD in older women
is warranted. The paper concludes with a discussion of assessment and
treatment options. doi:10.1300/J074v19n01_07 *[Article copies available for
a fee from The Haworth Document Delivery Service: 1-800-HAWORTH. E-mail
address: <docdelivery@haworthpress.com> Website: <http://www.HaworthPress.
com> © 2007 by The Haworth Press, Inc. All rights reserved.]*

KEYWORDS. Trauma, PTSD, women, aging, traumatic reactions

Since the 1980s, a vast research literature on posttraumatic stress disorder has developed, documenting acute and chronic traumatic reactions in civilian and non-civilian populations. Much is now known
regarding the nature of trauma and the prevalence of trauma reactions as
a common part of life experience. It is estimated that most Americans
will have at least one traumatic event in their lives and will recover
(Elliot & Briere, 1995). Furthermore, within the subset of the population that will develop PTSD, recovery in over half of the diagnosed
cases occurs within three months (American Psychiatric Association,
1994). Studies of trauma encompassing a broad spectrum of traumatic
events support this fact (Herman, 1989; Foa & Rothbaum, 1989; Kulka,
Schlenger, Fairbank, Hough, Jordan & Marmar, 1990). Though the
bulk of mental health research has reflected a more pathological view of
trauma (Bonanno, 2004; Kelley, 2005; Linley & Joseph, 2005), contemporary studies on resilience among Holocaust and other trauma survivors have posited that resilience and recovery from trauma may be
more normative (Bonanno, 2004; Brenner, 2005).

While recovery from trauma may be expected for most individuals, research studies reveal that special populations, especially those who have
had high, repeated exposure to trauma, are subject to chronic or complex
PTSD and warrant clinical attention (Herman, 1989; Foa & Rothbaum,
1989; Breslau, Davis, Andreski & Peterson, 1991; Walker, 1991). In this
regard, PTSD appears to be gender sensitive: approximately 8% of
American men but 20% of American women develop PTSD (Paige,
2003). Though men are more frequently exposed to various types of life
trauma events, women are subjected, more often, to crimes of repeated
sexual and physical assault which can result in prolonged PTSD symptoms. Recent research suggests that trauma and PTSD among certain
subpopulations of older women is likely to be underestimated (Higgins &

Follette, 2002). These women frequently present in medical and mental health settings with poor physical health and high levels of depression and anxiety which can mask trauma-related reactions and histories (Wolkenstein & Sterman, 1998). Though some formidable research studies now exist that examine trauma presentation among women receiving treatment in health-care settings and substance abuse programs, only a handful of studies are available that focus on the particular experiences of older women and PTSD. Much is not yet known regarding the life course of women with PTSD as they advance into later years, or of the developmental unfolding of specific female trauma populations, such as female Holocaust survivors (see Bernsten & Rubin, 2006). And, while there is a question regarding the degree to which experiences of older women differ from older men with trauma histories, the research literature nonetheless does offer special clinical considerations and recommendations regarding trauma and older women. To better understand the nature of PTSD among older women, it is first necessary to understand the nature of PTSD and trauma experience.

WHAT IS POSTTRAUMATIC STRESS DISORDER?

To meet the criteria of PTSD, an individual must be exposed to a traumatic event that evoked an actual or perceived threat to the person's life or physical integrity, and continues to elicit intense fear, horror and/or helplessness. Traumatic events can include combat, child abuse and neglect, terrorism, rape and sexual assault, motor vehicle accidents, disasters, community or domestic violence, captivity or torture. Traumas that can lead to development of PTSD can include any emotional state of discomfort or stress resulting from memories of an extraordinary catastrophic experience which shattered the survivor's sense of invulnerability. According to the Diagnostic and Statistical Manual of Mental Disorders (DSM-IV), PTSD is defined as an anxiety disorder which typically occurs three months following exposure (American Psychiatric Association, 1994). Though the traumatic event has passed, the individual is plagued with a cluster of symptoms which, in effect, keep the arousal, pain and heightened vulnerability of the trauma "alive." A founding father of trauma work, Abraham Kardiner (1941), observed that survivors act as if the trauma is still existent and enact protective behaviors which failed to protect them initially from trauma. Symptoms can center on reliving the traumatic event (e.g., recalling sensory and/or graphic details, intrusive images or memories, reoccurring nightmares and/or highly emotional panic states or flashbacks); avoiding reminders of the event by means of "numbing" behaviors (e.g., detaching from people associated with the event or from loved ones, avoiding places, people, activities associated with the event or loss of interest in everyday activities); and hyperarousal (e.g., being easily startled, difficulty concentrating or staying asleep, sudden irritability or outbursts of anger).

COURSE AND PREVALENCE OF PTSD

PTSD is one of a few diagnoses in the DSM-IV that identifies an environmental stressor as the salient cause of the psychological disturbance (deVries, 1996; Root, 1996). The diagnostic construct is based on data obtained on war veterans and on the psychological effects among women who were exposed to rape, sexual abuse and domestic violence (deVries, 1996; Root, 1996). Hence, it is one of the first diagnoses that provides a social historical context to suffering and is less descriptive of an intrinsic individual model of illness (deVries, 1996). Cultural factors naturally affect the course and recovery of PTSD. Numerous studies document the positive effects of social support that can correct the deleterious effects of trauma (deVries, 1996). Culture is crucial to how individuals cope with trauma, as it either provides a buffer that helps individuals heal or it may exacerbate stress factors as in the case of minorities who have experienced much isolation and stigma (deVries, 1996; Root, 1996). Though American women develop PTSD more frequently than American men, and older women appear to be under-diagnosed, it is difficult to discern how frequent PTSD occurs among older cohorts of women. Several researchers have found that older women do not typically disclose trauma (Higgins & Follette, 2002; Wolkenstein & Sterman, 1998), even though older women who present with depression and anxiety were identified in one study of mental health clinic populations as having complex histories of domestic and sexual trauma (Wolkenstein & Sterman, 1993). More studies are needed to estimate course and prevalence among older cohorts of American women.

IS GENDER A RISK FACTOR FOR PTSD?

Consistent in the research literature is the finding that women are more at risk for PTSD (Breslau, Davis, Andreski & Peterson, 1991;

Norris, 1992; Resnick, Kilpatrick, Dansky, Saunders & Best, 1993). This finding parallels reported rates for depression and other anxiety disorders among the population (Robins & Reiger, 1991). The higher prevalence of PTSD among women has been explained by the fact that women are more likely to experience repeated trauma and risk to body integrity, as in the case of physical or sexual assault (Kulka et al., 1990; Walker, 1991; Herman, 1992; Foa & Riggs, 1993; Turner & Lloyd, 1995; Higgins & Follette, 2002; Krause, Shaw & Cairney, 2004). Several authors have concluded that while American men are more likely to experience a traumatic event, American women are more likely to develop PTSD as they are prone to high rates of severe, sustained abuse (Walker, 1991; Herman, 1992; Courtois, 2004). Though prevalence rates differ among studies due to their methodologies, consensus exists that rates of PTSD in response to sexual assault are higher than those engendered from other trauma events, especially if revictimization has occurred. In fact, Kilpatrick et al. (1989) found rape to be the event most associated with lifetime PTSD (80%).

Though greater numbers of American women are at higher risk for developing PTSD than are their male counterparts, the relationship between gender and trauma is not well understood. Even less is known regarding the prevalence and nature of PTSD among older cohorts of American women (Saxe & Wolfe, 1999; Higgins & Follette, 2002; Krause, Shaw & Cairney, 2004). This is due, in part, to the fact that earlier trauma research and general health research in America typically examined the health of men, and not women. Though trauma is part of human history and life, the disciplined study of trauma by the medical and mental health professions focused on the experience of white males exclusively, specifically combat veterans (van der Kolk, McFarlane & Weisaeth, 1996). Reliable research on the female experience is also limited because earlier research relied on retrospective, self-report measures of perceived trauma that make comparison difficult across studies (Higgins & Follette, 2002; Krause, Shaw & Cairney, 2004).

PTSD among older adults, in particular, is not well understood. As Krause, Shaw and Cairney discern (2004), a majority of studies on trauma have focused on either children or young adults. When the experiences of older adults have been studied, it has been restricted either to a single traumatic event or involvement in combat. Studies addressing Holocaust survivors provide an important perspective (see Amir & Lev-Wiesel, 2003). At the same time, data obtained on studies of trauma and older adults have not been drawn from random samples making it difficult to generalize findings to the wider population of older adults (Norris, 1992). Most studies on older adults and trauma have tended to pool participants into one single group so that those participants aged 65 and older are treated as one cohort (Krause, Shaw & Cairney, 2004). As a consequence, when older adults are lumped together in a research sample, specific age cohort influences cannot be delineated and analyzed accordingly. As a consequence, the effects of significant historical realities that have shaped people's worldviews of suffering and coping options are embedded within the group as a whole and not by cohort (Krause, Shaw & Cairney, 2004).

Understanding trauma as a life span event is important because of its persistent impact on older adults. Yet, despite a proliferation of research on trauma, limited information exists regarding the frequency and impact of interpersonal trauma across the life span (Higgins & Follette, 2002; Krause, Shaw & Cairney, 2004). This finding is significant because the research literature suggests that women who are most likely to develop PTSD have been exposed to interpersonal violence and/or sexual abuse, have experienced repeated trauma, and are at risk for revictimization (Higgins & Follette, 2002; Saxe & Wolfe, 1999; Turner, 1995).

Other studies indicate a strong correlation between a history of interpersonal trauma and greater vulnerability or risk of illness and physical health problems in later life (Walker et al., 1992; Doron & Newton, 2000; Green & Schnurr, 2000; Frayne, Seaver, Loveland et al., 2004). A history of childhood sexual abuse or adult sexual assault has been found to correlate with higher levels of depression and PTSD in population samples (Tyra, 1993; Polusny & Follette, 1995). Rates of interpersonal trauma in older women are predicted to be high but difficult to prove (Higgins & Follette, 2000). Case studies of older men and women (deVries, 1996) suggest that older trauma survivors are at risk for an intensification of trauma symptoms or delayed trauma reactions when stressful life events occur (e.g., retirement, loss of social supports), with decreases in coping capacities. The following section presents an overview of the studies of older women and trauma to identify specific aspects, address clinical issues, and to suggest future research avenues.

RESEARCH ON OLDER WOMEN, TRAUMA AND IMPLICATIONS FOR TREATMENT

Despite being underrepresented as an area of trauma research, some studies have examined the relationship between trauma and older adults. In one study of older American men and women, three cohort groups were studied regarding the relationship between exposure to trauma over the life course and physical health status in later life (Krause, Shaw & Cairney, 2004). It was found that the young old (65-74), as compared to the old-old (74-84) and the oldest old (85 and over), were at greatest risk for poor health complications. This study is significant because it allows for a life course perspective and attempts to address whether the age of traumatic exposure is relevant to onset of poor health. These researchers surveyed a large sample of distinct elderly groups rather than joining all older subjects together, and assessed whether health at age 70, 80 or 85 is linked with traumatic events that arose earlier in life. The findings of this study support the hypothesis that cumulative exposure to trauma does erode health in later life–with respect to acute and chronic health conditions. In another study, Frayne et al. (2004) compared the frequency of medical symptoms and health among a large sample of women. Women with PTSD across the sample experienced more medical problems and poor physical health than women who reported depression alone or neither depression or PTSD (Frayne et al., 2004). In another study of the effects of trauma on older women, Higgins and Follette (2002) reported that women who experienced interpersonal trauma had more health problems than those who reported other traumatic histories.

In one of two studies on the effects of trauma on women later in life, Higgins and Follette (2002) examined the relationship between interpersonal trauma and its long-term impact upon the psychology and health of women over the age of 60. Their sample of women members were recruited from the community, the average age was 70, they were primarily Caucasian, and the majority were widowed or divorced/separated. Of significance, the authors utilized a semistructured interview format to assess specific histories of childhood sexual abuse, childhood physical abuse, and adolescent versus adult sexual victimization, in addition to self-report inventories to measure psychological and physical health. Researchers found that a majority of participants (71.6%) had experienced at least one type of interpersonal trauma, with domestic violence being the most common. A majority also reported two or more types of trauma which suggests that revictimization was a common experience (Higgins & Follette, 2002). Sexual assault in adulthood resulted in the highest stress rating among sample members. Of importance was the distinction of women who reported a history of multiple victimization associated with rape, childhood abuse and domestic violence which was associated with high levels of psychological and physiological distress.

These older women reported experiencing more avoidant behaviors, disturbed sleep, hypervigilance, anxiety, and depressive reactions which correlate with findings of other studies on younger women with similar trauma histories.

Higgins and Follette underscored the need to question older women about interpersonal trauma histories, particularly exposure to lifetime traumas. This point was echoed through the mental health literature (Wolkenstein & Sterman, 1998; Courtois, 2004) and is especially relevant to women in substance abuse programs (Fullilove, Fullilove, Smith, Winkler et al., 1993). Wolkenstein and Sterman (1998) examined this issue in their study of older women among two mental health clinic populations. They addressed how a high percentage of older women presenting with serious depression and anxiety symptoms later became identified as women with longstanding childhood and marital abuse histories. These women presented with serious, more "traditional" mental illness symptomatology and did not report earlier childhood and marital abuse at the time of admission, nor did intake procedures assess these factors. The authors found that earlier history of domestic violence and marital violence was very prevalent among older women, as were the adverse effects of trauma on their physical health. They suggested that what may have traditionally been perceived or diagnosed as persistent mental health disorders may in fact be some form of posttraumatic or abuse syndrome (Wolkenstein & Sterman, 1998). Courtois (2004) concurs and recommends that clinicians include questions about possible trauma, and also assess the presence of posttraumatic and/or dissociative symptomatology.

The implications for clinical practice and services to older adults are that trauma appears to be associated with adverse health effects. Therefore, it would appear crucial that information on exposure to trauma be obtained routinely during intake exams–both in medical and mental health settings. Since older adults are high users of health care, identifying and properly treating those with prolonged trauma histories may provide ways to reduce unnecessary or escalating medical costs (Krause, Shaw & Cairney, 2004). Moreover, medical staff and personnel involved in intake procedures and history-taking need to identify, assess and develop trauma sensitive skills, while learning to cope with the trauma histories of their patients (van der Kolk et al., 1996). Higgins and Follette (2002) suggest it would be beneficial to utilize an interdisciplinary team approach to assess trauma history with older women as they may not discuss their trauma experiences with any or all health-care providers. Finally, it should be noted that many women in the Higgins and Follette study were reportedly ashamed of their abuse histories. Many of these older women had never disclosed their abuse histories, having grown up in a time when disclosure was not an option.

ASSESSMENT

The first goal of assessment is to identify the presence of a traumatic history and to evaluate for PTSD. A "gold standard" in PTSD treatment is that clearly defined DSM-IV target symptoms must be present, since the experience of a trauma does not provide the basis for diagnosis of PTSD (Foa & Meadows, 1997). To complement one's clinical interview, many assessment tools are available to assess PTSD. Self-report measures include the PTSD Symptom Scale (Foa, Riggs, Dancu & Rothbaum, 1993; Foa et al., 1993). The Structured Clinical Interview is widely used to detect symptoms but is not a good indicator of symptom severity (Spitzer et al., 1990). Additional assessment tools to utilize include the Geriatric Depression Scale, a self-report measure of depression in older adults that possesses solid psychometric properties (Yesavage et al., 1983), and the Trauma Symptom Inventory which is particularly useful with older populations as it is designed to discern the level of trauma-related symptoms in adults that stem from childhood and adult exposure to trauma (Briere, Elliott & Harris, 1995). Finally, the Older Americans Resource and Services Center or OARS (Duke University Center for the Study of Aging, 1978) is a measure that assesses health problems, health functioning and use of medical service, and is highly relevant to older women.

TREATMENT OPTIONS

Multiple treatment modalities have been used to treat PTSD across populations. Consensus exists in the research literature that effective treatment of PTSD needs to follow specific phases that utilize different approaches within each (Herman, 1992; van der Kolk et al., 1996; Courtois, 2004). These phases should include: (1) a phase of stabilization in which education, validation of traumatic responses, and verbalization of feelings occur; (2) deconditioning of traumatic memories; (3) restructuring of traumatic personal beliefs; (4) reestablishment of secure social and interpersonal relationships; and (5) accumulation of restitutive emotional experiences (van der Kolk et al., 1996). Psychotherapy supplemented by psychopharmacology (to reduce depressive/anxiety symptoms) is a well-accepted standard of care (van der Kolk et al., 1996; Courtois, 2004).

Treatment outcome research supports the necessity of controlled exposure to traumatic memories. Several effective methods exist, including imaginal flooding; implosion therapy; desensitization; stress inoculation training; and a combination of cognitive reprocessing, education and exposure. Of these, imaginal flooding and implosion therapy have been found to sustain long-term symptomatic relief among rape survivors and Vietnam combat veterans (van der Kolk et al., 1996, 246). Eye Movement Desensitization and Reprocessing (EMDR) is a relatively new treatment that makes use of rapid eye movements while the patient recalls and maintains an image of the original traumatic experience. Though its effects have been reported to be very benefical for some PTSD patients, early outcome studies suffered from methodological weaknesses. More recent studies suggest EMDR is an effective treatment for reducing trauma symptoms in survivors of childhood sexual abuse (Wilson et al., 1995; Edmond, 2004).

A few authors have described individual clinical vignettes of treatment of older female survivors of trauma (Aarts & op den Velde, 1996; Lantz & Buchalter, 2003; Wolkenstein & Sterman, 1998). They tend to emphasize use of psychosocial interventions, including group support, cognitive behavioral therapy, and individual psychotherapy to facilitate coping with distressing feelings, memories and current life concerns (Lantz & Buchalter, 2003). For sleep disturbances, relaxation training and guided imagery are useful as well as promotion of social skills and management of anxiety (Courtois, 2004; Lantz & Buchalter, 2003). Cognitive behavioral treatments have been more subject to controlled outcome studies and have been the most rigorously tested (Foa & Meadows, 1997). In these therapy approaches, prolonged exposure and stress inoculation are central to obtaining reduction of PTSD symptoms for rape and sexual abuse survivors.

Psychodynamic treatments, either group or individual therapy, may offer benefits as well, but have not been effectively evaluated on a number of measures. As survivors of interpersonal violence often experience marked deficits in attachment and trust/safety issues, psychodynamic interventions are said to be helpful in addressing both conscious and unconscious reenactments of trauma. Psychodynamic interventions tend to focus on tasks of mourning losses, developing meaning to past and present experiences, facilitating acceptance of one's life, reestablishing self-coherence and awareness of self-continuity, and achieving increased ego integration (Aarts & op den Velde, 1996).

Wolkenstein and Sterman (1998) note several advantages of group treatment for older women with abuse histories. They argue that much education regarding the nature of violence and the consequences of living with violence in families and individuals can best be achieved in a group format. They contend that normalization of social rules and expectations within older cohort experiences of marriage can be maximized in group treatment. The group format also allows patients to build new relationships not based on shame and secrecy. They stress as well that the group treatment setting may be the only place the older woman can disclose a history of domestic violence.

Mind-body interventions may also be relevant to the treatment of trauma as many clients who suffer from complex interpersonal traumas are said to be alienated from their bodies and themselves. As Courtois (2004) indicates in her meta-analysis review of treatment for complex trauma, many of these clients are in a perpetual state of "disconnect." Mind-body techniques, such as guided imagery and hypnosis, appear to be effective and can be helpful in fostering a state of calm, positive self-soothing and improved affect regulation.

RECOMMENDATIONS FOR FUTURE RESEARCH

The number of women over the age of 60 will increase dramatically. Though many will not have experienced as much social censorship regarding disclosure of interpersonal violence as those in earlier studies, the impact of their trauma histories will continue to pose important considerations regarding the problems faced by women trauma survivors. Future research needs to include large-scale studies that survey broad samples of older females and focus specifically on their experience of trauma, PTSD treatment and the particular psychosocial needs of older women. Additionally, studies that are sensitive to ethnocultural variables are needed to discern rates of PTSD among minority women and to clarify whether significant differences exist. As issues of domestic violence and interpersonal trauma gain greater expression among the current generation of women, they will have more options available for coping with interpersonal trauma. It will become increasingly important for future researchers to assess this growing population of older women, and to identify their specific treatment needs.

REFERENCES

Aarts, P.G. & op den Velde, W. (1996). Prior traumatization and the process of aging: Theory and implications. In B. van der Kolk, B. McFarlane & L. Weisaeth (Eds.), *Traumatic stress: The effects of overwhelming experience on mind, body and society* (pp. 359-377). New York: Guilford Press.

American Psychiatric Association (APA) (1994). *Diagnostic and statistical manual of mental disorders* (4th ed.). Washington, DC: Author.

Amir, M. & Lev-Wiesel, R. (2003). Time does not heal all wounds: Quality of life and psychological distress of people who survived the Holocaust as children 35 years later. *Journal of Traumatic Stress, 16,* 295-299.

Bernsten, D. & Rubin, D.C. (2006). Flashbulb memories and posttraumatic stress reactions across the life span: Age-related effects on the German Occupation of Denmark during World War II. *Psychology and Aging, 21,* 127-139.

Bonanno, G.A. (2004). Loss, trauma, and human resilience: Have we underestimated the human capacity to thrive after extremely aversive events? *American Psychologist, 59*(1), 20-28.

Brenner, I. (2005). On genocidal persecution and resilience. *Mind and human interaction, 14,* 335-351.

Breslau, N., Davis, G.C., Andreski, P. & Peterson, E. (1991). Traumatic events and posttraumatic stress disorder in an urban population of young adults. *Archives of General Psychiatry, 48,* 216-222.

Briere, J., Elliott, D. & Harris, K. (1995). Trauma Symptom Inventory: Psychometrics and association with childhood and adult victimization in clinical samples. *Journal of Interpersonal Violence, 10*(4), 387-401.

Courtois, C.A. (2004). Complex trauma, complex reactions: Assessment and treatment. *Psychotherapy: Theory, research, practice, training, 41,* 412-425.

deVries, M.W. (1996). Trauma in cultural perspective. In B. van der Kolk, A. McFarlane & L. Weisaeth (Eds.), *Traumatic stress: The effects of overwhelming experience on mind, body and society* (pp. 398-413). New York: Guilford Press.

Doron, S. & Newton, T. (2000). Women and trauma: A clinical forum. *National Center for PTSD Clinical Quarterly, 9*(1), 9-10.

Duke University Center for the Study of Aging (1978). *Multidimensional Functional Assessment: The OARS methodology* (2nd ed.). North Carolina: Duke University.

Edmond, R. (2004). Assessing the long-term effects of EMDR: Results from an 18-month follow-up study with adult female survivors of CSA. *Journal of Child Sexual Abuse, 13*(1), 69-86.

Elliot, D.M. & Briere, J. (1995). Posttraumatic stress associated with delayed recall and sexual abuse: A general population study. *Journal of Traumatic Stress, 8*(4), 629-648.

Foa, E.B. & Meadows, E.A. (1997). Psychosocial treatments for posttraumatic stress disorder: A critical review. *Annual Review of Psychology, 48,* 449-80.

Foa, E.B. & Riggs, D.S. (1993). Post-traumatic stress disorder in rape victims. In J. Oldham, M. Riba & A. Tasman (Eds.), *American psychiatric press review of psychiatry* (Vol. 12, pp. 273-303). Washington, DC: American Psychiatric Press.

Foa, E.B., Riggs, D.S., Dancu, C.U. & Rothbaum, B.O. (1993). Reliability and validity of a brief instrument for assessing post-traumatic stress disorder. *Journal of Traumatic Stress*, 6, 459-474.

Foa, E.B., Rothbaum, B.O., Riggs, D.S. & Murdock, T.B. (1991). Treatment of posttraumatic stress disorder in rape victims: A comparison between cognitive behavioral procedures and counseling. *Journal of Consulting and Clinical Psychology*, 59(5), 715-723.

Frayne, S.M., Seaver, M.R., Loveland, S., Christiansen, C.L., Spiro III, A., Parker, V.A. & Skinner, K.M. (2004). Burden of medical illness in women with depression and posttraumatic stress disorder. *Archives of Internal Medicine*, 164(12), 1306-1312.

Fullilove, M., Fullilove, R., Smith, M., Winkler, K. et al. (1993). Violence, trauma, and post-traumatic stress disorder among women drug users. *Journal of Traumatic Stress*, 6(4), 533-543.

Green, B.L. & Schnurr, P.P. (Winter 2000). Trauma and physical health. *National Center for PTSD Clinical Quarterly*, 9(1), 1-5.

Herman, J. (1992). Complex PTSD: A syndrome in survivors of prolonged and repeated trauma. *Journal of Traumatic Stress*, 5, 377-391.

Higgins, A.B. & Follette, V.M. (2002). Frequency and impact of interpersonal trauma in older women. *Clinical Geropsychology*, 8(3), 215-226.

Kardiner, A. (1941). *The traumatic neuroses of war*. New York: Hoeber.

Kelley, T.M. (2005). Natural resilience and innate mental health. *American Psychologist*, 60(3), 265.

Kilkpatrick, D.G., Saunders, B.E., Amick-McMullan, A., Best, C.L.,Veronen, L. & Resnick, H.D. (1989). Victim and crime factors associated with the development of crime-related post-traumatic stress disorder. *Behavior Therapy*, 20, 199-214.

Krause, N., Shaw, B. & Cairney, J. (2004). A descriptive epidemiology of lifetime trauma and the physical health status of older women. *Psychology and Aging*, 10 (4), 637-648.

Krystal, H. (1981). Integration and self-healing in posttraumatic states. *Journal of Geriatric Psychiatry*, 14(2), 165-189.

Kulka, R.A., Schlenger, W.E., Fairbank, J.A., Hough, R.L., Jordan, B.K. & Marmar, C.R. (1990). *Trauma and the Vietnam War generation: Report of findings from the National Vietnam Veterans' Readjustment Study*. New York: Brunner/Mazel.

Lantz, M.S. & Buchalter, E.N. (April 2003). Posttraumatic stress disorder: When older adults are victims of severe trauma. *Clinical Geriatrics*, 11(4), 30-33.

Linley, A.P. & Joseph, S. (2005). The human capacity for growth through adversity. *American Psychologist*, 60(3), 262-264.

Norris, F.H. (1992). Epidemiology of trauma; Frequency and impact of different potentially traumatic events on different demographic groups. *Journal of Consulting and Clinical Psychology*, 60(3), 409-418.

Paige, Sr. (2003). Post-traumatic stress disorder (PTSD).emedicine.com. retrieved from *http://www.emedicinehealth.com/fulltext/29064.htm*

Polusny, M. & Follette, V. (1995). Long term correlates of child sexual abuse: Theory and review of the empirical literature. *Applied and Preventive Psychology,* 4, 143-166.

Rabasca, L. (1999). Women addicts vulnerable to trauma. *APA Monitor Online,* 30(2). *http:www.apa.org/monitor/feb99/women.html.*

Resnick, H.S., Kilpatrick, D.G., Dansky, B.S., Saunders, B.E. & Best, C.L. (1993). Prevalence of civilian trauma and posttraumatic stress disorder in a representative national sample of women. *Journal of Consulting and Clinical Psychology,* 61(6), 984-991.

Robins, L.N. & Reiger, D.A. (1991). *Psychiatric disorders in America: The Epidemiologic catchment area study.* New York: The Free Press.

Root, M. (1996). Women of color and traumatic stress in 'domestic captivity': Gender and race as disempowering statuses. In A. Marsella, M. Freidman, E. Gerrity & R. Scurfield (Eds.), *Ethnocultural aspects of posttraumatic stress disorder: Issues, research and clinical applications* (pp. 363-387). Washington, DC: The American Psychological Association.

Saxe, G. & Wolfe, J. (1999). Gender and posttraumatic stress disorder. In P. Saigh & D. Bremner (Eds.), *Posttraumatic stress disorder, A comprehensive text* (pp. 160-179). Needham Heights, MA: Allyn & Bacon.

Schnurr, P.P. (Summer 1996). Trauma, PTSD, and physical health. *PTSD Research Quarterly,* 7(3), 1-7.

Schumm, J.A., Hobfoll, S.E. & Keogh, N.J. (2004). Revictimization and interpersonal resource loss predicts PTSD among women in substance-use treatment. *Journal of Traumatic Stress,* 17(2), 173-181.

Shmotkin, D., Blumstein, T., & Modan, B. (April 2003). Tracing long-term effects of trauma: A broad-scope view of Holocaust survivors in late life. *Journal of Consulting and Clinical Psychology,* 71(2), 223-234.

Spitzer, R.L., Williams, J.B., Gibbon, M. & First, M.B. (1990). *Structured clinical interview for DSM-III-R, Patient Edition.* New York: Biometrics Department, New York State Psychiatric Institute.

Turner, R.J. & Lloyd, D.A. (1995). Lifetime traumas and mental health: The significance of cumulative adversity. *Journal of Health and Social Behavior,* 36, 360-376.

Tyra, P. (1993). Older women: Victims of rape. *Journal of Gerontological Nursing,* 19, 7-12.

van der Kolk, B., McFarlane, A. & van der Hart, O. (1996). A general approach to treatment of posttraumatic stress disorder. In B. van der Kolk, A. McFarlane & L. Weisaeth (Eds.), *Traumatic stress: The effects of overwhelming experience on mind, body and society* (pp. 417-440). New York: Guilford Press.

Walker, L.E. (1991). Posttraumatic stress disorder in women: Diagnosis and treatment of battered woman syndrome. *Psychotherapy,* 28, 21-29.

Wilson, J.P., Friedman, M.J. & Lindy, J.D. (2001). *Treating psychological trauma and PTSD.* New York: Guilford Press.

Wolkenstein, B.H. & Sterman, L. (1998). Unmet needs of older women in a clinic population: The discovery of possible long-term sequelae of domestic violence. *Professional Psychology: Research and Practice,* 29(4), 341-348.

Yehuda, R. & McFarlane, A.C. (1995). The conflict between current knowledge about PTSD and its original conceptual basis. *Americal Journal of Psychiatry,* 152, 1705-1713.

Yesavage, J., Brink, T., Rose, T., Lum, O., Huang, V., Adey, M. & Leirer, V. (1983). Development and validation of a geriatric depression screening scale: A preliminary report. *Journal of Psychometric Research,* 17, 34-39.

For More Information: Weblinks

National Center for PTSD
National Institute of Mental Health
International Society for Traumatic Stress Studies
National Center for PTSD of the Department of Veterans Affairs
Posttraumatic Stress Disorder Alliance, Posttraumatic Stress Disorder Resource Center

doi:10.1300/J074v19n01_07

The Older Female Patient with a Complex Chronic Dissociative Disorder

Richard P. Kluft, MD

SUMMARY. Dissociative disorders are rarely considered in the diagnostic assessment of older women, despite the fact that the existence, appearance and characteristics of certain dissociative disorders in older populations have been known and described since the 1980s. This communication reviews the core phenomena of Dissociative Identity Disorder and related forms of Dissociative Disorder Not Otherwise Specified, the natural history of their phenomena from youth to old age, and describes common presentations of dissociative disorders in older women. It also reviews the treatment of complex chronic dissociative disorders and discusses alternative approaches to their psychotherapy in the older female patient. It is crucial to recognize and respect the importance of appreciating individual differences among older dissociative patients and to individualize their treatments accordingly. doi:10.1300/J074v19n01_08 *[Article copies available for a fee from The Haworth Document Delivery Service: 1-800-HAWORTH. E-mail address: <docdelivery@haworthpress.com> Website: <http://www.HaworthPress.com> © 2007 by The Haworth Press, Inc. All rights reserved.]*

KEYWORDS. Dissociation, multiple personality disorder, women, aging, DID, MPD

Address correspondence to: Richard P. Kluft, MD, 111 Presidential Blvd., Suite 238, Bala Cynwyd, PA 19004 (E-mail: rpkluft@aol.com).

[Haworth co-indexing entry note]: "The Older Female Patient with a Complex Chronic Dissociative Disorder." Kluft, Richard P. Co-published simultaneously in *Journal of Women & Aging* (The Haworth Press, Inc.) Vol. 19, No. 1/2, 2007, pp. 119-137; and: *Mental Health Issues of Older Women: A Comprehensive Review for Health Care Professionals* (ed: Victor J. Malatesta) The Haworth Press, Inc., 2007, pp. 119-137. Single or multiple copies of this article are available for a fee from The Haworth Document Delivery Service [1-800-HAWORTH, 9:00 a.m. - 5:00 p.m. (EST). E-mail address: docdelivery@haworthpress.com].

OVERVIEW

The dissociative disorders include Dissociative Amnesia, Dissociative Fugue, Depersonalization Disorder, Dissociative Identity Disorder, and a spectrum of conditions related to these entities categorized under Dissociative Disorder Not Otherwise Specified. The dissociative disorders are typically diagnosed in younger patients and rarely diagnosed for the first time in older populations. Their true incidence and prevalence among older individuals is unknown. Memory difficulties and wandering and personality changes in older populations usually are assumed to be due to organic causes (e.g., organic mental syndromes, the impact of physical disease, the side effects of medications) or attributed to more well-known mental disorders. Furthermore, there is a minimal index of suspicion for dissociative disorders among clinicians who specialize in the care of older populations.

Yet dissociative symptoms are prominent among the sequelae of trauma (Koopman, Classen, & Spiegel, 1994), and older populations are by no means immune from traumatic events. Their medical conditions, accidents, and injuries may expose them to overwhelming experiences, they may be vulnerable to victimization by all manner of predators (including their families and those entrusted with their care), and they may be differentially more affected by disasters than younger populations (Shinfuku, 2005).

Often the factors noted above lead clinicians to overlook, misunderstand, or misdiagnose posttraumatic and dissociative phenomena. While some dissociative disorders are generally (but not always) time-limited events that tend toward remission, such as dissociative amnesia and dissociative fugue, many cases of depersonalization disorder become chronic or recurrent, and Dissociative Identity Disorder may wax and wane, but is generally chronic unless interrupted by successful treatment. While most cases of posttraumatic stress disorder remit or respond to treatment within months or years, a considerable minority remain chronic and refractory. Such patients may retain their posttraumatic symptoms, including dissociative phenomena, into their older years. (For an overview of trauma responses, see Kluft, Bloom, & Kinzie, 2000.)

This contribution will focus on Dissociative Identity Disorder (hereafter DID) and related forms of Dissociative Disorder Not Otherwise Specified (hereafter DDNOS) in older female populations. These forms of dissociative disorder are most commonly found in women, and are likely, in the absence of successful treatment, to persist into their older years (Kluft, 1985). Since the distinctions between DID and many cases of DDNOS are difficult to draw, and most cases of DID spend most of their adult lives giving the appearance of DDNOS (Kluft, 1985), hereafter I will often use DID to encompass both conditions.

DID AND DDNOS

Prevalence

Many recent studies from North America, Europe, and Asia (summarized in Kluft, 1999a & 2005; Ross, 1997) demonstrate that when psychiatric patient populations are systematically screened, previously undiscovered DID can be diagnosed in 0.5-5% of those psychiatric inpatients studied, and in even higher percentages of patients in day hospitals for the treatment of drug abuse. In epidemiological studies of normal North American populations, about 1% endorse the symptoms of DID in structured interviews (Ross, 1991, 1997). On clinical assessment, about half appear to have clinical dissociative disorders.

Given that one can expect previously undiagnosed DID to be present in between one in 20 and one in 200 psychiatric patients, and for there to be an even higher prevalence of dissociative disorders in general, it seems reasonable to consider the possibility of dissociative disorders in the assessment of virtually any psychiatric patient. Given that females outnumber males in most series at ratios between 5:1 and 9:1 (Kluft, 1991; Putnam et al., 1986), and that female longevity exceeds male life expectancy, it becomes especially important to raise it as a consideration in evaluating female patients, especially in patients beyond early middle age.

DSM-IV Diagnostic Criteria, Description, Natural History, and Course

The diagnostic criteria for DID are listed in Table 1, and the subtypes of DDNOS that are related to DID are listed in Table 2. These disorders are "the delivery and maintenance system for achieving an intrapsychic multiple reality disorder, the purpose of which is the patient's internal effort to carry on with the semblance of a normal life when contending with life's actual realities has proven impossible" (Kluft, 1998, 1999a; Kluft, 2005, p. 634). To preserve the hope of safety and the notion that crucial relationships are or can become positive and loving, the over-

TABLE 1. DSM-IV Diagnostic Criteria for Dissociative Identity Disorder

A. The presence of one or more distinct identities or personality states (each with its own relatively enduring pattern of perceiving, relating to, and thinking about the environment and self).
B. At least two of these identities or personality states recurrently take control of the person's behavior.
C. Inability to recall important personal information that is too extensive to be explained by ordinary forgetfulness.
D. The disturbance is not due to the direct physiological effects of a substance (e.g., blackouts or chaotic behavior during alcohol intoxication) or a general medical condition (e.g., complex partial seizures). Note: in children, the symptoms are not attributable to imaginary playmates or other fantasy play.

(Reprinted with permission from the *Diagnostic and Statistical Manual of Mental Disorders*, Fourth Edition (Copyright 2000). American Psychiatric Association.)

TABLE 2. Dissociative Disorder Not Otherwise Specified

This category is included for disorders in which the predominant feature is a dissociative symptom (i.e., a disruption in the usually integrated functions of consciousness, memory, identity, or perception of the environment) that does not meet the diagnostic criteria for any specific Dissociative Disorder. Examples include:
1. Clinical presentations similar to Dissociative Identity Disorder that fail to meet full criteria for this disorder. Examples include presentations in which a) there are not two or more distinct personality states, or b) amnesia for important personal information does not occur.

[Description and example 1.]
(Reprinted with permission from the *Diagnostic and Statistical Manual of Mental Disorders*, Fourth Edition (Copyright 2000). American Psychiatric Association.)

whelmed child "develops ingenious and resourceful fantasies that undo or modify what the mind cannot accept. An aspect of this adaptation is the development of alternate identities and selves that act in accordance with these adaptive fantasies" (Kluft, 2005, p. 634). These alters are guided by concepts of goodness and safety that were understood to best protect the child from further danger and harm. As a rule, these concepts are masochistic and reflect a sense of needing to submit to powerful others in order to be safe.

The manifestations of the alters are often quite subtle. Although the DSM diagnostic criteria themselves would seem to suggest that DID should have overt and dramatic symptoms, overt switches are far less common than alters' influencing one another from behind the scenes (Kluft, 1985). Kluft (2005) has introduced the term "dissociative surface" to encompass observable and inferable phenomena associated with the alters' impacts upon the alter ostensibly in executive control of the body and mind.

The alters often interact among themselves in an inner world that re-capitulates the interactions among the patient and the significant others during the patient's childhood. Those suffering DID must be understood to participate in and partake of three realities (Kluft, 1998) that often overlap and/or intrude into one another. The first is historical reality, perceived as accurately as possible, but subject to distortions and misperceptions. The second is historical reality as memories of that reality become modified and revised by distortions, fantasies, misperceptions, transferences, projections, misinformation, post-event infuences, and contaminations. The third involves events enacted in the inner world of the alters, which may intrude into the patient's awareness and be misperceived as events that actually are occurring or have occurred in historical reality (Kluft, 1999a). These realizations position the clinician to listen more sensitively to the often puzzling, contradictory, and difficult-to-assess representations made by many DID patients. While some may actually occur in their contemporary lives, some may prove to be flashbacks mistaken for contemporary events, and some may prove to be events involving an alter or alters representing past abusers and an alter or alters representing the patient, usually as a child, in the inner world, or the "third reality" (Kluft, 1998).

DID and related forms of DDNOS are characterized by lesions or problems of identity, memory, thinking, containment, and cohesive conation as well as difficulties with the switching process (Kluft, 1999a). Lesions of identity may include the presence of alters, states of depersonalization, absence of identity, confusion about identity, and the impingement of one or more alters on another or the combined co-presence of two or more alters.

Lesions of memory "may include amnesia for past events, blocks of lost contemporary time, uncertainty about whether certain events have or have not occurred, fragmentary recall of traumata, and the experience of events as dream-like or derealized and of uncertain veracity. There may also be a variety of amnestic barriers across the alters, which may be aware of one another, unaware of one another, or have directional amnesia (e.g., alter A knows about alter B and is aware of its thoughts and activities, while alter B knows little or nothing about A, is unaware of A's thoughts, and is amnestic when A has executive control)" (Kluft, 1999a, p. 3).

Lesions of thinking involve those failures of reasoning that stem from defensive distortions of reality, child-like and magical notions of problem resolution and assuring one's safety, disavowals of crucial information, and prioritizing considerations of the inner world of the alters over considerations based on contemporary reality. DID patients, who may be intellectually gifted and capable of impressive achievements in areas that do not touch on their painful issues, are nonetheless capable of convincing themselves of the rightness of positions drawn from their experiences and understandings of trauma that are logically preposterous and potentially self-destructive.

Lesions of containment encompass the intrusion of one or more alters into another and the leakage of the memories, feelings, and sensations of one alter into the awareness and experience of another alter. This includes a patient's becoming aware of the voices and actions of other alters, experienced as hallucinations or "made actions" (Kluft, 1987). Lesions of cohesive conation are problems with the distribution of executive control across alters. "Alters' sense of control of themselves and their actions is often compromised, as is their sense of ownership, responsibility, and voluntary control over choices and actions" (Kluft, 1999a, p. 4). Lesions of the switch process occur when the process of switching is not smooth, leading to jarring or incomplete transitions, or when switching is occurring with such frequency and/or rapidity that the person cannot achieve continuity in what he or she is attempting to accomplish.

Etiology of DID and Related Forms of DDNOS

A comprehensive review of the many theories of the etiology of DID is beyond the scope of this article. At present there are two major competing theories of etiology for such conditions, summarized in Kluft (1999a).

In brief, the first holds that these conditions are chronic dissociative adaptations developed after exposure to overwhelming life experiences during childhood in individuals with high hypnotic talent (e.g., Kluft, 1984; Putnam, 1989; Ross, 1997). In support of this are data demonstrating the high hypnotizability of this patient cohort (Frischholz et al., 1992), studies demonstrating that 95% of children and adolescents with dissociative disorders have documented abuse (Coons, 1994; Hornstein & Putnam, 1992), and that many recovered memories of abuse reported by DID patients have been documented (Kluft, 1995, 1998).

The second holds that these conditions are iatrogenic social-psychological artifacts induced by therapists and maintained by suggestible patients. In support of this are data demonstrating that many phenomena of DID can be induced transiently by suggestive techniques in laboratory settings (e.g., Spanos, 1996).

Despite the furor that often surrounds this debate, the demonstration of a single unequivocal rather than merely alleged/accused DID case of iatrogenic etiology has yet to occur. This is important because those convinced it is iatrogenic usually point to the mere existence of cases of DID as proof of their perspective, assuming the iatrogenic etiology a priori. Furthermore, a demonstration that DID could be created iatrogenically would not rule out the possibility of its naturalistic occurrence.

A careful review of the literature reveals that although cases of DID can become more complex and develop more alters in response to iatrogenic influences, and although it is possible if not probable that some cases of DDNOS have been "promoted" to fulfilling full DID criteria by iatrogenic influences (some of which are epiphenomena of completely appropriate interventions), there is no proof that completely normal individuals can be caused to have DID through iatrogenic influences (Kluft, 1999a). It remains conceivable that phenomena close to DID can be created by non-therapeutic interventions for covert military/espionage purposes under unusual circumstances with little resemblance to therapy settings (e.g., Estabrooks, 1957; Ross, 2000).

The Natural History of DID

The natural history of DID reveals its close connection with certain forms of DDNOS (Kluft, 1985). Six percent of DID patients demonstrate florid DID symptoms on an ongoing basis. The remaining 94% spend the majority of their lives manifesting phenomena that would yield a diagnosis of DDNOS or no dissociative disorder at all under most circumstances, unless they are temporarily decompensated, dropping their defenses in treatment, or interviewed in a manner that elicits their longitudinal experiences of dissociative phenomenology. This is done in the Structured Clinical Interview for the Diagnosis of DSM-IV Dissociative Disorders-Revised (SCID-D-R) (Steinberg, 1994). Fourteen percent remain overtly DID but disguise their condition with remarkable facility unless their adaptation is overwhelmed by intercurrent stressors or unique triggers. Most DID patients, 80%, instead have "windows of diagnosability" during which their DID is overt and easily recognized. These windows are usually associated with psychosocial stress, but may be triggered by anniversaries of abuse or loss or by potent signifiers or reminders of past abuses. Once a DID patient has been diagnosed and begins to participate in a treatment that addresses this condition, his or her customary more hidden adaptation is chronically destabilized, leading to more frequent overtness and the appearance that the patient is "getting worse in psychotherapy."

DID is a disorder of childhood onset. Instances of alleged adult onset have been reported, but these reports are rare, and have been disputed. It is thought to emerge in the context of overwhelming experiences, usually but not exclusively associated with child abuse. There has been a general agreement that persons who first experience overwhelming experiences after age eight or nine are not likely to develop DID (Kluft, 1984a, 1984b).

A study of the natural history of DID allows certain admittedly oversimplified generalizations about the condition's presentations across different age groups (Kluft, 1985). Most dissociative children rapidly learn to disguise or contain most of their alters, but direct and indirect manifestations of their alters, amnesia or distraction may be noted, such as denied out-of-character behavior, forgetfulness, day-dreaming, and being perceived as liars. Adolescents with DID/DDNOS might show aggressive tendencies (mostly males) or chaotic adolescent turmoil or make quiet withdrawn presentations. Children and adolescents with DID are rarely diagnosed as such. Among adults, those diagnosed in their 20s often are fairly out of control with open psychopathology suggesting borderline personality disorder, psychosis, substance abuse, or bipolar disorders. Those diagnosed in their 30s, the most common cohort, often present as depressed, anxious, controlled, and mildly obsessional. Those diagnosed in their 40s often were individuals of considerable strength and attainment, whose psychopathology was well-hidden. Often a desperate sense that time was passing and their appreciation that they were having more and more trouble containing themselves brought them for treatment.

Those diagnosed from their 50s through their 90s include a minority with florid manifestations that were either missed or kept well-hidden, but most had a single alter that was out the vast majority of the time. On exploration it was found that many personalities had atrophied, gone dormant, or had not taken over for years. This has been called the "one alter predominant presentation." These findings, though anecdotal, are buttressed by the fact that in Kluft's "natural history" project, all of the patients diagnosed with DID while younger, but who remained untreated, demonstrated a much changed presentation in their "second look" evaluations a decade or more later. Almost all of those reassessed at ages greater than 60 had all undergone a metamorphosis to a "one alter predominant" presentation.

The older patients with DID generally presented with symptoms of anxiety and depression, and were found to have first rank symptoms and inner voices without signs of a chronic psychotic disorder. Following up these phenomena had led to the DID diagnosis. This is illustrated by a recent case.

Case Example. A 74-year-old mental health professional in part-time practice was referred for medical hypnosis for chronic pain. She also had severe anxiety and depression. She hoped that hypnosis could help with these as well, because she was intolerant of psychotropic medications. She announced that she had been in treatment for over 40 years with over 30 therapists, but continued to suffer. She gave a bland history. Her high score on the Hypnotic Induction Profile (Spiegel & Spiegel, 1978), a measure of hypnotizability, indicated she was a good candidate for hypnosis. In her first hypnotic session she entered trance readily, and manifested many hypnotic phenomena. She achieved considerable pain relief. In the next session she either could not or would not enter trance. In the subsequent session I tried to help her explore the events of the previous session. She revealed that she had not gone along with me in order to see how I would react to her not performing, and not being obedient. I wondered what would cause her such concerns, because no historical material suggested a basis for it. We explored her prior treatments. Almost universally, one or more good sessions had raised her hopes, which had been dashed when the initial promise of the treatment dissolved rapidly into mutual frustration. I speculated that there must be some motivation at work more powerful than the wish to recover–perhaps there were things from which she needed to protect herself, and there was fear that a successful treatment might expose her to them. She found herself nodding "yes" without knowing why. I speculated that there might be a part of the mind that was a quick learner, a part that in the interests of such protection, figured out where therapy might be going and stifled her participation in treatment. In response, the patient looked startled, and reported an inner voice saying (to the patient) "You couldn't handle knowing." When I inquired, the patient revealed that she had never wanted to admit that she had been the victim of father-daughter incest and other forms of severe abuse. The inner voice revealed that while there were several other parts, only she (apart from the host, who had presented for treatment) had remained active in recent years, an inner guardian of the secrets and a buffer against emotional pain. This part revealed that it was having an increasingly difficult time keeping painful memories at bay, and the physical discomfort associated with those memories was, in the form of body memories, causing the patient's pain syndromes. It advised the patient to remain in treatment with me, "because I can't help you anymore the way I used to be able to help you."

The Impact of Aging on DID Psychopathology

The relationship between aging and DID psychopathology is both intricate and complex. On the average, DID patients receive this diagnosis in their early 30s after spending 6.8 years in the mental health-care delivery system with 3.4 other diagnoses (Putnam et al., 1986). Therefore, while DID is almost invariably of childhood onset, it usually is only diagnosed in early middle adulthood. Its manifestations may either remain unchanged or undergo transitions over time. One characteristic alteration, the muting of DID manifestations over time, may, by becoming more covert, give the appearance that the condition had gone into remission over the years.

My own approach to classifying older DID patients is to distinguish among those (1) grown old, (2) diagnosed old, (3) relapsed secondary to abuse or triggers while old, and (4) destabilized by comorbidity while old.

DID patients grown old includes those who have been diagnosed with DID and allied forms of DDNOS during or prior to their adult lives. They either were not treated or their treatments did not lead to the cure of their conditions. Many have become more muted in their presentations, with the atrophy and/or inactivation of many alters and/or the withdrawal of many alters into an inner world. Other DID patients retain all or most of their alters, but the alters rarely if ever emerge, and they exert their influence upon the alter that is in apparent executive control from behind the scenes. These are forms of the "one alter predominant" presentation described in older DID patients by Kluft (1985).

It is often unclear whether such changes are responses to these DID patients' lives being less traumatic and/or less likely to bring them into situations that might mobilize alters (such as sexual activity), to enhanced non-dissociative coping with maturity, to cognitive declines that make dissociative barriers more difficult to maintain, or to reduced hypnotizability with aging. In many cases it is clear that several or all of these factors are at play. Such patients must be treated with an awareness that their dissociative barriers may give way suddenly and thereafter may be incapable of being reconstituted. Ironically, if such a patient abruptly becomes aware of the voices of alters, is flooded with flashbacks or dysphoria, or begins to make accusations against those the patient feels have wronged him or her, an involutional or late onset form of psychosis may be diagnosed.

Some DID patients do not appear to undergo these changes, and retain a typical adult form of DID into their older years. Such individuals usually show no signs of major illness or cognitive decline despite their advanced years. Usually they have had treatments that were very helpful, but which were not pursued to complete integration.

Those diagnosed old include DID patients who had never entered the mental health-care delivery system, those who were misdiagnosed in earlier evaluations and those whose disorders were so well-contained earlier in life that it is only as their dissociative barriers fray and/or are further stressed that they can become aware of and able to report the symptoms that raise the index of suspicion for a dissociative disorder. Some of these previously contained individuals had spent their entire adult lives as caretakers, often for one or more individuals who had abused them. At times the terminal illness or death of an abuser triggers recollections of mistreatment, precipitating a combination of delayed posttraumatic stress disorder and DID symptomatology.

Assessment

The diagnosis and differential diagnosis of DID can be challenging enterprises. Both have been summarized in a recent review (Kluft, 2005). Routine mental status examinations and commonly-employed psychological batteries usually do not make major contributions. They do not adequately assess relevant areas of inquiry, and often lead to false negative diagnoses. The study of the dissociative disorders is a new field, and its discoveries are not represented in instruments and examinations developed prior to the field's growth and maturation.

Many scales and interviews are now available (Kluft, 2005), but it is not likely that they will be utilized absent an index of suspicion that a dissociative disorder might be present. Clinicians who are unfamiliar with the clinical presentations of dissociative disorders will do best if they supplement their evaluations with inquiries about suggestive signs of DID (e.g., Kluft, 2005) or items from a special mental status examination for chronic complex dissociative disorders (Loewenstein, 1991). A list of suggestive signs appears as Table 3. Most items are self-explanatory, but clinicians are often perplexed by items 12 and 14. It is possible to elicit phenomena that are not alters, but instead are either transient ego states or responses based on an effort to please the inter-

TABLE 3. Suggestive Signs of DID (and Related Forms of DDNOS)

1. Prior treatment failure
2. Three or more prior diagnoses
3. Concurrent psychiatric and somatic symptoms
4. Fluctuating symptoms and levels of function
5. Severe headaches and other pain syndromes
6. Time distortions, time lapses, or frank amnesia
7. Being told of unremembered behaviors
8. Others noting observable changes
9. The discovery of objects, productions, or handwriting in one's possession that one cannot account for or recognize
10. Hearing voices (80% or more within the head) that are experienced as separate, often urging the patient toward some activity
11. The patient using "we" in a collective sense or making self-referential statements in the third person
12. The eliciting of other entities through hypnosis or a drug-facilitated interview
13. A history of child abuse
14. An inability to recall childhood events from ages 6 to 11

(Kluft, 1991, 2005)
(Reprinted with permission from the *Annual Review of Psychiatry* (Copyright 1991). American Psychiatric Association.) (Reprinted with permission from SLACK Incorporated: Kluft, R.P. (2005). Diagnosing dissociative identity disorder. *Psychiatric Annals*, *35*(8), 633-643.)

viewer or a misunderstanding of the inquiry. Actual alters have senses of their identity, self-representations, autobiographical memories, and a sense of ownership of their own thoughts and actions. Also, while amnesia for early childhood is normal, amnesia for one's elementary school years is less common, raising the suspicion of dissociation during childhood.

Loewenstein's (1991) special mental status is a rich source for questions about major areas of DID phenomenology: (1) indications of the DID process at work (e.g., differences in behavior, linguistic indications, switching/shifting); (2) sign of the patient's high hypnotic potential (e.g., enthrallment, trance logic, out-of-body experiences); (3) amnesia; (4) somatoform symptoms; (5) posttraumatic stress disorder symptoms; and (6) affective symptoms.

A range of useful diagnostic instruments is noted in a recent review (Kluft, 2005). For routine use, it is helpful to be familiar with one screening instrument and one structured diagnostic interview. The Dissociative Experiences Scale (Bernstein & Putnam, 1986) asks the subject to score his or her subjective perception of what percentage of time 28 dissociative phenomena are experienced on a scale from 0-100%. Although not all DID patients score 30 or more, scores of 30 or more are much more associated with dissociative disorders than lower scores, and suggest a need for further evaluation. The Structured Clinical Interview for DSM-IV Dissociative Disorders–Revised (SCID-D-R) (Steinberg, 1994) allows for an in-depth study of a patient's experience of five groups of dissociative phenomena (amnesia, depersonalization, derealization, identity confusion, identity alteration) scored on a scale of 1 through 4, summarized in a total score between 5 and 20. Normal subjects generally score under 8, groups of mixed psychiatric patients average scores of 8-12. Scores above 12 are not commonly found in psychiatric patients without pathological dissociation; scores of 15 or more are usually associated with clinical dissociative disorders; DID patients who are not being defensive often score 17-20. The SCID-D-R also allows assessment of associated phenomena, detailed follow-ups of positive answers and a section for clinical observations. This combination often allows the clinician to make a firm dissociative disorder diagnosis.

Treatment Recommendation

The treatment of DID and related forms follows the three-stage pattern of trauma treatment described by Herman (1992). A phase of *safety* during which the patient receives sanctuary and support and is strengthened is followed by a phase of *remembrance and mourning* during which the mind's representation of its traumatic experiences is explored, processed and mastered, and during which the consequences of the traumas and their sequelae are grieved. The mind is reintegrated, the impact of the experiences upon one's identity and sense of self is addressed, and disrupted development, functions, and roles are resumed in a final phase of *reconnection*.

In DID/DDNOS, however, it is useful to envision a more complex model, the components of which are listed in Table 4. Stages 1-3 generally correspond to Herman's stage of safety; stage 4 corresponds to Herman's stage of remembrance and mourning; and stages 5-9 correspond to Herman's stage of reconnection. In practice these stages are far from precise, and blend into one another. Furthermore, some alters may already have integrated before others are discovered, so that the overall treatment is often a mosaic of the concerns of different stages at any one point in time. In addition, while complete integration is a definitive outcome, many patients choose or can go no farther than to bring about a better situation among the alter personalities, an outcome called resolution (Kluft, 1991, 1993).

TABLE 4. The Stages of Treatment for DID/DDNOS

1. Establishing the psychotherapy
2. Preliminary interventions
3. History gathering and mapping
4. Metabolism of the trauma
5. Working toward integration/resolution
6. Integration/resolution
7. Learning new coping skills
8. Solidification of gains and working through
9. Follow-up

(Kluft, 1991)
(Reprinted with permission from the *Annual Review of Psychiatry* (Copyright 1991). American Psychiatric Association.)

The treatment of DID is a complex matter, best described in specialized texts and reviews (e.g., Kluft, 1999b; Kluft & Fine, 1993; Putnam, 1989; Ross, 1997). However, many special considerations apply to the treatment of older patients (Kluft, 1988). The treatment of DID can be prolonged, painful, and arduous. It may pose unacceptable or insurmountable medical and psychological risks to vulnerable patients. When physical resilience and ego strengths are compromised, it can be very difficult for a DID/DDNOS patient to tolerate and contain such challenging and frequently rigorous regimens. When dissociative barriers are being breached, it can be difficult for a patient with compromised strengths to contain him or herself between sessions. A supportive or partial treatment may be much more workable (Kluft, 1999b).

Therefore, in working with the older dissociative patient, the clinician begins treatment hoping to bring about a resolution, which is a stable improvement based on achieving a more functional and facile communication, cooperation and collaboration among the alters that remain separate. Often a good resolution involves the integration of some, but not all, of the alters. Complete definitive integration is often achieved in relatively strong DID patients with less complex alter systems, but is not a realistic goal in the treatment of most of the more compromised and complex among older DID/DDNOS patients.

It becomes important to treat each patient with an awareness of and sensitivity to the nuances of her unique situation. Often the best (theoretical) treatment for the condition is not the best treatment for the patient. Such issues and concerns should be discussed with the patient. The patient's own preferences and priorities should be respected whenever feasible and possible. Sometimes concerned others should be consulted, but with caution. Unfortunately, most concerned others immediately jump to the conclusion that the older patient should be spared all pain associated with a difficult treatment. Sometimes this reflects genuine concern, but often it reflects a wishful avoidant stance motivated to minimize inconvenience, expense, the possible impact of painful family secrets upon themselves, relationships and reputations, etc. A not uncommon situation occurs when an older person begins to contend with abuse by one of her own parents, who is known to her children only as a beloved grandparent. Often the patient's children, who have been affected by the patient's psychopathology and impairment, and saw their grandparents as a refuge from their parents' chaotic home, assume the DID patient is deranged, telling falsehoods, or making excuses for their failings. They may discount the DID patient's statements about her experiences and treat her in an unsympathetic manner.

It has been my experience that most older DID patients have spent years bewildered by what has become of their lives. They have spent decades dwelling in confusion and uncertainty about aspects of their identity and personal history, confused and ashamed about their symptoms and ways of handling situations and relationships. Achieving a further sense of clarity, more solidification of their identities, and greater comprehension of their circumstances has given them more peace of mind than they had achieved in decades of running from their own memories. This positions them to approach their remaining years well-grounded, more accepting and forgiving of themselves, and with some degree of comfort, equanimity, and peace of mind. On the basis of this experience, it has seemed useful to help older DID patients who are motivated for treatment and can give informed consent.

It is also useful to bear in mind that since most dissociative barriers gradually fray with advancing age, the hoped-for goal of avoiding certain pains forever is rarely accomplished. I have seen older DID patients who either were not diagnosed until their dissociative barriers weakened, or who resisted exploration until it was forced upon them by their diminishing capacities to keep material out of awareness. These unfortunate individuals were flooded with terribly ego-dystonic memories and affects at a point in their lives at which the resources for containment available in most therapies were beyond the capacities of their diminished ego strengths and cognitive capacities. In my clinical experience it has seemed wiser to help older DID patients who are motivated to better understand their situations while they still have the resources to do so. Of course, those who decide against this course of action should not be pressured or criticized. It is important to get informed consent for either course of action.

In treating the older female patient with DID, treatment should be paced carefully and gently. Work with traumatic material should be done in the least unsettling manner possible, employing more vigorous techniques only when the traumatic material continues to generate unsettling symptoms despite its being processed conversationally. When abreaction proves necessary, it should be approached with the less disruptive fractionated abreaction technique (Fine, 1991, 1993; Kluft, 1990), which was designed to protect older and more fragile patients from more vigorous classic abreactions and exposure/flooding models, and supported with the temporizing techniques (Kluft, 1989) developed to stabilize patients between sessions.

The treatment should strive more to reduce the intrusive power of painful material than to resolve it completely, prioritizing the patient's safety, stability, and quality of life over a more thorough and theoretically more desirable processing. With an older population, the theoretical and practical differences between long-term and short-term therapeutic goals and results often are collapsed and indistinct. This having been said, there are some older patients for whom a more definitive processing will be necessary in order to resolve their difficulties.

In dealing with patients more acutely aware of the finite limitations of their lives, pressing for integration, which alters often insist on perceiving as their deaths, becomes a minor consideration. In younger patients years of discussion and negotiation may be necessary to bring about an understanding of integration and an appreciation of its value. With older patients a major investment in such efforts is neither helpful nor pragmatic. If alters integrate spontaneously after discussing/processing their issues, or if they request help in integrating after dealing with their concerns, such processes should be accepted and encouraged. When one encounters staunch opposition or strong apprehension about integration in an older patient, the clinician should honor these misgivings unless the clinician becomes convinced that they are being used to prohibit work on matters that must be addressed in order for the patient to be helped toward greater comfort and function.

RESOURCES FOR FURTHER STUDY

There are relatively few resources for those interested specifically in the treatment of dissociative disorders in older female patients. The experience of the last several decades has demonstrated that clinicians who try to treat dissociative patients within the paradigms with which they are familiar, but fail to learn the specifics of dissociative disorder treatment generally, fail to provide effective and/or definitive treatment for this group of patients (Kluft, 1985, 1993).

Those interested in learning more should consult texts that are considered classics in the dissociative disorders field (e.g., Kluft & Fine, 1993; Putnam, 1989; Ross, 1997); explore the Website of the International Society for the Study of Dissociation (www.issd.org) which includes its treatment guidelines; consult the classic treatment articles from *DISSOCIATION* (archived on line at http://libweb.uoregon.edu/news/stories/dissociation.htm), and articles in the successor to *DISSOCIATION*, *The Journal of Trauma and Dissociation.*

Workshops on the treatment of dissociative disorders are given both nationally, locally, and online by the International Society for the Study of Dissociation. However, when all is said and done, the best resource for the clinician who needs answers quickly is consultation with colleagues experienced with this patient population.

NEED FOR ADDITIONAL RESEARCH

The dissociative disorders have been heavily debated and lightly researched. They are controversial in many quarters, and their prevalence and importance have not been recognized and prioritized by most governmental and non-governmental funding sources. Since research often "follows the money," there has been little systematic research on most of the basic and crucial issues in the study of these patients and their treatment. It has been notoriously difficult to obtain grant funding in these areas, and there are no strong signs that this situation is improving. Progress in the dissociative disorders continues to be made by dedicated clinicians whose contributions often remain anecdotal or quite limited in terms of their ability to generate data suitable for statistical analysis, and by academicians who "piggy-back" the study of dissociative patients onto other projects and provide instructive and thought-provoking, but still somewhat obstructed, views and insights into an important but still largely unstudied domain of both mind and brain.

REFERENCES

American Psychiatric Association (2000). *Diagnostic and statistical manual of mental disorders, Fourth Editon–Text Revision.* Washington, DC: American Psychiatric Association.

Bernstein, E., & Putnam, F.W. (1986). Development, reliability, and validity of a dissociation scale. *Journal of Nervous and Mental Disease*, 174, 727-734.

Coons, P.M. (1994). Confirmation of childhood abuse in child and adolescent cases of multiple personality disorder and dissociative disorder not otherwise specified. *Journal of Nervous and Mental Disease*, 182, 461-464.

Estabrooks, G.H. (1957). *Hypnotism, revised edition*. New York: Dutton..

Fine, C.G. (1991). Treatment stabilization and crisis prevention: Pacing the therapy of the multiple personality disorder patient. *Psychiatric Clinics of North America*, 14, 661-675.

Fine, C.G. (1993). A tactical integrationalist perspective on the treatment of multiple personality disorder. In R.P. Kluft & C.G. Fine (Eds.), *Clinical perspectives on multiple personality disorder* (pp. 135-153). Washington, DC: American Psychiatric Press.

Frischholz, E., Lipman, L.S., Braun, B.G., & Sachs, R.G. (1992). Psychopathology, hypnotizability, and dissociation. *American Journal of Psychiatry*, 149, 1521-1525.

Herman, J. (1992). *Trauma and recovery*. New York: Basic Books.

Hornstein, N., & Putnam, F.W. (1992). Clinical phenomenology of child and adolescent multiple personality disorder. *Journal of the American Academy of Child and Adolescent Psychiatry*, 31, 1055-1077.

Kluft, R.P. (1984a). Treatment of multiple personality disorder. *Psychiatric Clinics of North America*, 7, 9-29.

Kluft, R.P. (1984b). Multiple personality in childhood. *Psychiatric Clinics of North America*, 7, 121-134.

Kluft, R.P. (1985). The natural history of multiple personality disorder. In R.P. Kluft (Ed.), *Childhood antecedents of multiple personality* (pp. 197-238). Washington, DC: American Psychiatric Press.

Kluft, R.P. (1987). First rank symptoms as diagnostic indicators of multiple personality disorder. *American Journal of Psychiatry*, 144, 293-298.

Kluft, R.P. (1988). On treating the older patient with multiple personality disorder: Race against time or make haste slowly? *American Journal of Clinical Hypnosis*, 30, 257-266.

Kluft, R.P. (1989). Playing for time: Temporizing techniques in the treatment of multiple personality disorder. *American Journal of Clinical Hypnosis*, 32, 90-98.

Kluft, R.P. (1990). The fractionated abreaction technique. In C. Hammond (Ed.), *Handbook of hypnotic suggestions and metaphors* (pp. 527-528). New York: Norton.

Kluft, R.P. (1991). Multiple personality disorder. In A. Tasman & S. Goldfinger (Eds.), *Annual review of psychiatry, Vol. 10* (pp. 161-188). Washington, DC: American Psychiatric Press.

Kluft, R.P. (1993). Treatment of dissociative disorder patients: An overview of discoveries, successes, and failures. *Dissociation*, 6, 87-101.

Kluft, R.P. (1995). The confirmation and disconfirmation of memories of abuse in multiple personality disorder: A naturalistic clinical study. *Dissociation*, 8, 253-258.

Kluft, R.P. (1998). Reflections on the traumatic memories of dissociative identity disorder patients. In S. Lynn & K. McConkey (Eds.), *Truth in memory* (pp. 304- 322). New York: Guilford.

Kluft, R.P. (1999a). Currrent issues in dissociative identity disorder. *Journal of Practical Psychiatry and Behavioral Health*, 5, 3-19.

Kluft, R.P. (1999b). An overview of the psychotherapy of dissociative identity disorder. *American Journal of Psychotherapy*, 53, 289-319.

Kluft, R.P. (2005). Diagnosing dissociative identity disorder. *Psychiatric Annals*, 35, 633-643.

Kluft, R.P., Bloom, S.L., & Kinzie, J.D. (2000). Treating traumatized patients and victims of violence. In C. Bell (Ed.), *Psychiatric aspects of violence: Issues in prevention and treatment* (pp. 79-102). San Francisco: Jossey-Bass.

Kluft, R.P., & Fine, C.G. (Eds.) (1993). *Clinical perspectives on multiple personality disorder*. Washington, DC: American Psychiatric Press.

Koopman, C., Classen, C., & Spiegel, D. (1994). Predictors of posttraumatic stress symptoms among survivors of the Oakland/Berkeley, California firestorm. *American Journal of Psychiatry*, 151, 888-894.

Loewenstein, R.J. (1991). An office mental status examination for complex chronic dissociative symptoms and multiple personality disorder. *Psychiatric Clinics of North America*, 14, 567-604.

Putnam, F. (1989). *Diagnosis and treatment of multiple personality disorder*. New York: Guilford.

Putnam, F.W., Guroff, J.J., Silberman, E.K., Barban, L., & Post (1986). The clinical phenomenology of multiple personality disorder. *Journal of Clinical Psychiatry*, 47, 285-293.

Ross, C. (1991). Epidemiology of multiple personality disorder and dissociation. *Psychiatric Clinics of North America*, 14, 503-518.

Ross, C. (1997). *Dissociative identity disorder: Diagnosis, clinical features, and treatment of multiple personality disorder*. New York: Wiley.

Ross, C. (2000). *Bluebird: Deliberate creation of multiple personality by psychiatrists*. Richardson, TX: Manitou Communications, Inc.

Shinfuku, N. (2005). The experience of the Kobe earthquake. In J. Lopez-Ibor, G. Christodoulou, M. Maj, N. Sartorius, & A. Okasha (Eds.), *Disasters and mental health*. Chichester, UK: John Wiley & Sons, Ltd.

Spanos, N. (1996). *Multiple identities and false memories: A sociocognitive perspective*. Washington, DC: American Psychological Association.

Spiegel, H., & Spiegel, D. (1978). *Trance and treatment: Clinical uses of hypnosis*. New York: Basic Books.

Steinberg, M. (1994). *Stuctured Clinical Interview for the Diagnosis of DSM-IV Dissociative Disorders–Revised*. Washington, DC: American Psychiatric Press.

doi:10.1300/J074v19n01_08

Sexual Problems, Women and Aging: An Overview

Victor J. Malatesta, PhD

SUMMARY. Expression of one's sexuality is a fundamental mental health need of all individuals, regardless of age and gender. While the popularity and widespread use of Viagra and similar medications for male erectile dysfunction have helped many individuals, it has also reinforced a more male-dominated view of sexuality–one that focuses more on genital function, and less on the relationship and issues of intimacy and meaning. Highlighting important issues and recent trends, the paper provides an overview of the diagnosis, description, etiology, assessment and treatment of women's sexual problems. A broad perspective on sexuality is emphasized, along with an understanding of the sexual response cycle. A selected review of the literature on older women and sexual dysfunction shows wide variability and the important role of biomedical, health and relational factors. In working with the sexual needs of older women, any therapeutic intervention should be based upon a solid understanding of the myths and realities of the sexual aging process, a keen understanding of the sexual challenges faced by older women, and a respect for the continuity of one's sexual lifestyle. doi:10.1300/J074v19n01_09 *[Article copies available for a fee from The Haworth Document Delivery Service: 1-800-HAWORTH. E-mail address:*

Address correspondence to: Victor J. Malatesta, PhD, 300 E. Lancaster Ave., Suite 207, Wynnewood, PA 19096.

[Haworth co-indexing entry note]: "Sexual Problems, Women and Aging: An Overview." Malatesta, Victor J. Co-published simultaneously in *Journal of Women & Aging* (The Haworth Press, Inc.) Vol. 19, No. 1/2, 2007, pp. 139-154; and: *Mental Health Issues of Older Women: A Comprehensive Review for Health Care Professionals* (ed: Victor J. Malatesta) The Haworth Press, Inc., 2007, pp. 139-154. Single or multiple copies of this article are available for a fee from The Haworth Document Delivery Service [1-800-HAWORTH, 9:00 a.m. - 5:00 p.m. (EST). E-mail address: docdelivery@haworthpress.com].

<docdelivery@haworthpress.com> Website: <http://www.HaworthPress.com>
© 2007 by The Haworth Press, Inc. All rights reserved.]

KEYWORDS. Sexuality, aging, women, dysfunction, sexual desire, arousal, orgasm

INTRODUCTION

Expression of one's sexuality is a fundamental mental health need of all individuals, regardless of age and gender. Compared to other aspects of mental health, however, human sexuality has been a relatively understudied area of scientific and clinical investigation. This deficiency is especially true with respect to the sexuality of older adults. While research and clinical studies over the last 30 years have helped to dispel the myth that the later years are sexless (as I noted in the *Journal of Women & Aging* in 1989), a range of societal and attitudinal misconceptions continues to interfere with the ability and inclination of many older adults to address their sexual needs.

A second area of deficiency relates to the fact that knowledge of women's sexuality and female sexual activity still lags seriously behind that of male sexuality (Everaerd & Laan, 2000). Although the popularity and widespread use of sildenafil (Viagra) and similar medications for male erectile dysfunction have been helpful to many individuals, it has also (1) resulted in the "medicalization" of sex therapy (with correspondingly less focus on psychosocial and interpersonal therapies for sexual problems); (2) de-emphasized the importance and primary role of the relationship; and (3) has unwittingly reinforced the traditional male-dominated view of sexual activity (i.e., penile-vaginal intercourse). This view has tended to emphasize sexual "function" over sexual intimacy and "meaning" (see Basson, 2000; Kaschak & Tiefer, 2002; Tiefer, 2001). Finally, while the scientific search for a female version of Viagra continues to elude pharmacologic researchers, there is serious concern that these efforts are misguided and misdirected.

These inadequacies and misconceptions come at a time when a recent comprehensive review of female sexual dysfunction has revealed a complex relationship between a woman's age and the presence of sexual dysfunction (West, Vinikoor, & Zolnoun, 2004). In eight of their reviewed studies, sexual dysfunction increased with age, while no relationship with age was reported in three studies. Other research has shown that four out of 10 women and nearly one-third of men report some type of sexual problem (Laumann, Paik, & Rosen, 1999). This work has indicated that sexual dysfunctions are a major public health problem that deserves increased study, identification, and treatment. To respond to this challenge, the U.S. Surgeon General in his recent Call to Action has emphasized the importance of sexual health across the life span, and its close relationship with physical and mental health (Office of the Surgeon General, 2001).

With these points in mind, the purpose of this paper is to address the sexual problems and related concerns of older women. Highlighting important issues and recent trends, the paper provides an overview of the diagnosis, description, etiology, assessment and treatment of women's sexual problems. The emphasis of this paper does not necessarily assume a heterosexual orientation. While there is an even greater need for research on lesbianism, homosexuality and other sexual minorities, some have argued that the general research is applicable because there is considerable overlap between heterosexual and homosexual behavior (Sadock, 1995). While this point is debatable, the interested reader is referred to the following sources for additional study: Dolan, 2005; Rose, 2002. Finally, as clinicians, we emphasize the importance of a thorough understanding of both "normal" and diverse sexualities as a prerequisite for studying, evaluating and treating sexual problems (Malatesta & Adams, 2001).

DEFINING SEXUALITY

Human sexuality is diverse and encompasses a complex and multifaceted set of biological, psychological, and sociocultural variables. An individual's sexuality includes everything ranging from one's genitalia, hormones, and basic sex drive, to sexual response, feelings, gender identity, and body image. In addition, unlike many forms of human behavior, one's sexuality and sexual activity are typically expressed within a relational and intimate interpersonal context. The interactive nature of human sexuality introduces additional variables, including communication, partner satisfaction, meaning and the ability to negotiate intimate relationships. Finally, individual sexuality is enmeshed with one's developmental and learning history, in addition to personality, mood state, and the culture in which one lives.

When this multitude of factors is superimposed upon normal individual differences in conjunction with one's unique pattern of aging and life experience, the result can be stated as a fact: *Variability (i.e., Diver-*

sity) of sexual expression increases with age. Thus, as is true of other aspects of the aging process, the sexual needs and behaviors of older adults are not easily categorized, and instead are quite diverse and differ markedly among individuals–whether heterosexual, homosexual, highly sexual, or sexually inactive (see Butler, 2000; Blumberg, 2003; Siegel & Schrimshaw, 2003).

Even though there is greater understanding and awareness of sexual diversity, there remains a strong, ingrained belief that heterosexuality is limited to or equated with sexual intercourse. This is a lingering societal myth that one's sexuality can only be expressed "in the bed" through sexual intercourse. Adherence to this myth limits our understanding and appreciation for the possibilities associated with sexuality in the later years. This myth may be particularly damaging for older adults for whom physical infirmity, being unpartnered, or residence in an assisted living or nursing home have seriously curtailed the opportunities for expression of sexual needs.

In contrast, a growing number of clinicians and researchers are emphasizing a broader perspective on human sexuality–one that incorporates not only the pioneering and revolutionary work of Masters and Johnson, Kaplan, and other writers, but also the recent studies of more feminist investigators, including Tiefer (2001, 2004), and Basson and her colleagues (Basson, 2000; Basson et al., 2003). Their work has emphasized the role of relational aspects of sexuality, social and cultural variation, issues of choice, and positive compensations for physical disability and illness. At the same time, their work has de-emphasized the importance of "correct genital performance," while focusing attention on the need to understand sexual activity in long-term relationships and how it differs from that experienced in the first 1-2 years of a heterosexual or homosexual relationship. Not surprisingly, this work has special applicability to the sexual concerns of older women.

While current psychiatric diagnosis of female sexual problems does not incorporate this broader perspective, it is still a necessary starting point. It also provides a foundation from which to think about and address a more sensitive framework.

MODELS OF SEXUAL RESPONSE AND THE DSM-IV-TR DIAGNOSIS OF SEXUAL PROBLEMS

Human sexual behavior has been viewed as the most sensitive of the biological response systems because it is functionally responsive to an array of physiological, cognitive-behavioral, and psychosocial-relational variables (Adams, 1981). Important early work included the development of testable and clinically useful models of sexual response, including Masters and Johnson's (1966, 1970) sexual response cycle (arousal, plateau [excitement], orgasm & resolution), and Kaplan's important inclusion of a desire phase. Although criticized as being more characteristic of men, the sexual response cycle was an important development that spurred an incredible amount of research and clinical activity. The Diagnostic and Statistical Manual of Mental Disorder, 4th Edition, Text Revision (DSM-IV-TR: American Psychiatric Association, 2000) continues to borrow heavily from the work of Masters and Johnson, and Kaplan, and utilizes a four-stage model to diagnose "sexual dysfunction." In this regard, sexual dysfunction is defined as a disturbance in the processes that characterize the sexual response cycle or by pain associated with sexual intercourse. The sexual response cycle is divided into the following four phases:

1. *Desire*: This phase consists of thoughts and fantasies about sexual activity and an interest or inclination to be sexual.
2. *Excitement*: This phase reflects both a subjective sense of pleasure and the accompanying physiological changes associated with sexual arousal (in the male: penile tumescence and erection; in the female: vasocongestion in the pelvis, vaginal lubrication and swelling of the external genitalia).
3. *Orgasm*: This phase reflects a peaking of sexual pleasure, with release of sexual tension and rhythmic contraction of the perineal muscles and reproductive organs.
4. *Resolution*: This phase consists of a sense of muscular relaxation and general well-being. During this phase, males are physiologically refractory to further erection and orgasm for a variable length of time that increases with age, while women show variability, may experience no refractory phase, and are able to respond quickly to additional stimulation. For these reasons, the refractory phase appears to have minimal relevance to women.

The DSM-IV-TR notes that "disorders of sexual response" can occur at any one or more of the phases. Thus, for women as well as men, sexual problems are classified in DSM-IV-TR into four major areas: (1) sexual desire disorders; (2) sexual arousal disorders; (3) orgasmic disorders; and (4) sexual pain disorders. A disorder in one category may lead to difficulties in another area. Additional categories include sexual dysfunction that is *due to a general medical condition*, and *substance-induced* sexual dysfunction. It should be noted that, unlike the male sexual response cycle, for women there may not be a clear progression from desire to arousal and orgasm. Female sexual response may also change over the reproductive lifecycle, including the menstrual cycle, pregnancy, the postpartum period, and menopause. These variations are a normal part of the female life cycle and are not reflective of psychopathology (West et al., 2004).

For accurate diagnosis, the DSM-IV-TR requires both an impairment in desire or objective performance *and* an indication that the disturbance causes marked distress or interpersonal difficulty. Therefore, it is possible that an individual may have a deficiency in a phase of sexual response, but not be distressed by it–personally or interpersonally. In this case, the individual would not meet full diagnostic criteria for a sexual dysfunction. This finding is particularly relevant for older adults and older women who typically show a great variability of response that is superimposed upon developmental milestones (e.g., menopause), illness, relational status, living situation, and other variables. Relatedly, the DSM-IV-TR describes "subtypes" of sexual dysfunction to address the onset, context, and etiological factors associated with a sexual dysfunction. Thus, sexual dysfunctions can be subtyped as either *Lifelong* or *Acquired, Generalized* or *Situational,* or either *Due to Psychological Factors* or *Due to Combined Factors.*

DESCRIPTION AND PREVALENCE

Sexual Desire Disorders

Although there has been an evolution in the description and classification of sexual desire disorders, there is no universally accepted definition (DeLamater & Sill, 2005). In DSM-IV-TR, *Hypoactive Sexual Desire Disorder* (HSDD) refers to a persistent and recurrent deficiency or absence in sexual thoughts, fantasies, and inclination to engage in sexual activity. Judgment of a "deficiency" or absence must take into account factors that affect sexual activity, including age and context of the person's life. The deficiency must also cause marked distress or interpersonal difficulty to qualify for the diagnosis. The diagnosis is also not made if the lack of sexual desire is the primary result of a medical condition or a substance. In that case, the diagnosis would include the qualifier of sexual dysfunction *due to a medical condition* or *substance induced.*

With respect to prevalence, converging evidence shows that complaints of low or absent sexual desire are one of the most common sexual dysfunctions in community and clinical samples alike. Earlier studies reflected prevalence estimates that ranged from 15-55%, and more recent cross-sectional studies show that increasing age is associated with decreased sexual desire (Laumann et al., 1999)–but not always so (see West et al., 2004). Moreover, DeLamater and Sill (2005) reported in their study of 745 women that "it is not until age 75 or older that the majority of women and almost a majority of men report a low level of sexual desire" (p. 147). In their large survey study of *Sex in America*, Michael et al. (1994) reported that "the dearth of sex among older women reflects the logistics of the marketplace for sexual partners, the higher mortality rate for men, and the value that women place on affection and continuity in sexual relations. It is not the desire but opportunity and attitude that make the difference for men and women" (p. 122). West et al. (2004) reported in their review of multiple studies that low sexual desire in women was associated with longer partner duration, partner dissatisfaction, many children, and financial concerns. Finally, in a large multiethnic study of 3262 midlife women, 40% reported a low frequency of sexual desire (Cain et al., 2003).

Sexual Aversion Disorder (SAD) is a relatively recent diagnostic category of sexual desire problems. SAD goes beyond low desire and avoidance of sexual activity to include sexual panic, sexual repugnance, and sexual phobia. Very little is known about the prevalence and etiology of SAD. Consistent with other clinical researchers, Masters, Johnson and Kolodny (1994) reported that SAD involves women two to three times more frequently clinically than men. However, it is unclear if SAD actually reflects a gender difference or is a function of other factors (e.g., a result of sexual trauma).

Sexual Arousal Disorders

In the DSM-IV-TR, *Female Sexual Arousal Disorder* (FSAD) is defined as a persistent or recurrent inability to attain or maintain an "adequate lubrication-swelling response of sexual excitement" until completion of sexual activity. This category has been criticized extensively with respect to women. A revision was recommended by an international consensus panel because of the omission of a subjective or "mental" component to women's view of sexual arousal. "Women mainly are speaking of mental excitement when they speak of sexual arousal" (Basson et al., 2000, pp. 56-57). Similarly, it was pointed out that women do not tend to focus on genital changes (i.e., vaginal lubrication) as a measure of arousal.

The category FSAD may be particularly inappropriate for older women for whom an attenuation of the lubrication-swelling response is completely normal–particularly for those who are post-menopausal and/or in long-term relationships. With respect to prevalence data, Heiman (2002) reported that there were minimal prevalence data for FSAD, and that it is rarely identified clinically as separate from either desire or orgasmic difficulties. West et al.'s (2004) review identified 12 studies that addressed arousal-excitement difficulties. Prevalence of female arousal disorder ranged from 20% to 30%, and in two studies, it increased with age. These latter findings in particular may be artifacts of other factors noted above.

Orgasmic Disorders

Female Orgasmic Disorder (FOD) is defined as a persistent or recurrent delay in, or absence of, orgasm following a "normal excitement phase." The DSM-IV-TR recognizes that there is wide variability in a woman's orgasmic response and that diagnosis of (FOD) must take this into account. To qualify for the diagnosis, the woman must also complain of "marked distress or interpersonal difficulty" associated with orgasmic difficulty. The international consensus panel pointed out that while some women typify Masters and Johnson's "mountain" of orgasmic release, often it is not representative of women's arousal and release under various circumstances (Basson et al., 2000). It was also reported that clinically at least five different orgasmic patterns may be identified and that these patterns changed from occasion to occasion. Finally, it should be noted that while orgasmic capacity increases with a woman's age, there is a generalized reduction in the physiological intensity of orgasmic expression (Masters & Johnson, 1966; see also Meston, Levin, Sipski et al., 2004).

The DSM-IV-TR (2000) also indicates that the capacity to experience orgasm increases with age and that FOD is more common in younger women. West et al. (2004) reported that prevalence data for orgasmic disorder ranged from below 20% to 30-40% in their review. They pointed out that women with diabetes were at greater risk for

FOD, as were those who engaged less frequently in sexual activity or had more conservative attitudes toward sexuality.

Sexual Pain Disorders

There are two major types of sexual pain disorders in women, dyspareunia and vaginismus. Dyspareunia is recurrent and persistent pain during intercourse. It is a prevalent condition that occurs at 10-21% in community samples and particularly in younger women (Laumann et al., 1999). West et al. (2004) found that prevalence of dyspareunia ranged from 0.9% to 75%, with bimodal frequencies of less than 10%. They hypothesized that the bimodal nature of the rates reflected many factors, such as the woman's age and reproductive status, and methodological issues. Laumann and colleagues (1999) found that coital pain differed by age, with the greatest likelihood of pain in the 18-29 year age group (21%), decreasing to an average of 14% in the 30- 49 year age group, and 8% in those 50-59 years old.

Vaginismus, an involuntary spasm of the vaginal musculature that interferes with intercourse, is a relatively rare disorder without concurrent dyspareunia (Heiman, 2002). Vaginismus can range from severe cases where penile and tampon insertion into the vagina is impossible because of the spasm and constriction. At the other end of the continuum, vaginismus may occur only partially or situationally. Presence of vaginismus should alert the clinician to assess for a history of sexual trauma.

ETIOLOGY OF SEXUAL PROBLEMS

A multivariate perspective is crucial in appreciating the causal complexity and variability of problems in sexuality. Sexual dysfunctions in general are caused by an interplay of biological and psychosocial factors. For instance, female desire difficulties have emphasized hormonal and relational factors, whereas sexual trauma has been associated with a range of sexual problems in many women as well as men (Malatesta & Adams, 2001; West et al., 2004). Longitudinal data have shown that although advancing age per se may be related to quantitative but not qualitative changes in sexual activity (George & Weiler, 1981), a host of variables that accompany the aging process may exert significantly adverse effects on sexual desire and activity, including: (1) physical illness and chronic disease; (2) medications and alcohol abuse; (3) relational and emotional problems, especially depression; (4) partner availability;

(5) sociocultural, family and personal expectations; and (6) a previous lifestyle of low sexual activity. This section will briefly highlight special topics of relevance to older women.

Disease and Illness

Sexual dysfunctions are often related to illness and disease. There may be an interaction between physical and secondary factors, ranging from a predominantly physical causation (e.g., cervical cancer) to a medical etiology with significant psychological sequelae. For example, while gynecologic cancer survivors show improvement in life areas, such as mood and social adjustment, 50% experience sexual difficulties that do not resolve (see Andersen, Woods, & Copeland, 1997). Other studies showed that while 27% of women with Type I diabetes reported sexual dysfunction, it was not associated with age, and many described marital difficulties. Depression was also a complicating factor, and more women with Type 2 diabetes displayed difficulties across the sexual response cycle, including complaints of vaginal discomfort (see West et al., 2004). Additional information regarding women, sexual problems, and biomedical disorders, including chronic pain, interstitial cystitis, breast cancer, and spinal cord injury, is provided in Malatesta and Adams (2001) and Schover and Jensen (1988).

Natural and Surgical Menopause

This is a complex area that reflects methodological concerns. Many studies have not addressed how ovarian function might influence the presence or absence of sexual dysfunction (West et al., 2004). While the general conclusion is that arousal problems, including lubrication insufficiency, tend to increase with age and progression through the perimenopausal transition, the question of desire difficulties is more difficult to answer because of multiple factors, including health and relationship quality. In their review, West et al. (2004) reported that the rate of reduced sexual desire was highest in naturally menopausal women, followed by surgically menopausal females who had an oophorectomy and perimenopausal women. They also noted one study that found, when controlling for age, level of sexual desire in menopausal women was not related to age, but to biological factors. Finally, West et al. reported that the predictors of orgasmic difficulty in menopausal women included age, vaginal dryness, recent bladder infection, depression, and bilateral oophorectomy (see also Dennerstein, Alexander, & Kotz, 2003).

Medications and Alcohol Use/Abuse

Multiple studies show that a vast array of drugs can interfere with any phase of female sexual response, including (1) selective serotonin re-uptake inhibitors (SSRIs); (2) heterocyclic antidepressants; (3) dopamine-blocking agents; (4) antihypertensive drugs; and (5) narcotics and sedative hypnotics, which decrease central nervous system (CSN) cortical activity (see Hendrick & Gitlin, 2004; Montgomery, Baldwin, & Riley, 2002). Alcohol, another CNS depressant, has been shown to affect sexual arousal and orgasm in women (Malatesta, Pollack, Crotty, & Peacock, 1982), and female alcohol abusers describe dysfunctions across the sequence of sexual response (see Wilsnack, 1991). More information is needed with respect to older women, sexual response, and alcohol and medication effects.

Depression and Body Image

Although there is a sizeable literature on the role of depression and sexual dysfunction, it is unclear whether depression is exerting its influence via biochemical substrates, lowered self-esteem, loss of pleasure and sensual awareness, or other factors. Many studies have also confounded depression with medication effects. Sexual desire and arousal problems and orgasmic difficulty are a common response to depression (Masters et al., 1994; West et al., 2004). Less is known about older women in this area.

With respect to body image, Koch et al. (2005) found that among their study of midlife women, the more a woman perceived herself as less attractive than when younger, the more likely she was to report a decline in sexual desire or frequency of sexual activity. Conversely, the more she perceived herself as attractive, the more likely she was to experience higher levels of sexual desire, orgasm, enjoyment or frequency of sexual activity. As important, self-perceived attractiveness did not depend on menopausal status (see also Tiggerman & Lynch, 2002). Finally, it is not surprising that body image concerns are especially challenging in the aftermath of breast cancer (see Anllo, 2000).

A Note on Sexual Inactivity

The issue of sexual inactivity is an understudied area that may reflect a different type of myth and misconception associated with aging and sexuality. It has been argued and generally assumed that extended periods of sexual inactivity may exert a physiological handicap (i.e., "use it or lose it") for older women and men who may or may not wish to engage in sexual activity at a later time. There are minimal data to substantiate this claim (Schover & Jensen, 1988), and it is unfortunate if this belief places unnecessary pressure on older adults. For many adults, sexual activity is a non-issue that must be respected and validated. Finally, it should be noted that older unpartnered women, who are not sexually active, tend to meet their sexual and affectional needs through a range of "nonsexual" activities–many of which may be viewed as compensatory (Malatesta, Chambless, Pollock, & Cantor, 1988).

ASSESSMENT AND TREATMENT ISSUES

Assessment and treatment of sexual dysfunction typically involves referral to a clinician or "sex therapist" who is a psychologist, psychiatrist, psychiatric social worker or nurse practitioner who possesses not only customary credentials and training in their respective fields, but also specialty training and experience in sexual assessment and sex therapy. The American Association of Sex Educators, Counselors and Therapists (AASECT) provides a certification program in sex therapy. It should also be noted that essentially all sex therapists have extensive training and experience in couples therapy–particularly since much of sex therapy involves a "blending" and integration of sex therapy procedures with couples therapy techniques (Malatesta & Adams, 2001).

Assessment of sexual problems typically addresses four distinct, but interrelated components, including (1) biomedical and health status; (2) the phases of sexual response; (3) individual psychological makeup, including personality, developmental liabilities, and mood state variables; and (4) interpersonal issues, relationship status, and partner variables, including ethnocultural and religious influences.

From multiple perspectives (ethical, evaluative and therapeutic), a case of sexual dysfunction remains outside of the domain of the mental health professional until biomedical factors have been addressed by medical personnel. The medical work-up represents an essential prerequisite for assessment of sexual dysfunction and also reflects the need for a working relationship with a specialist physician (e.g., gynecologist). This relationship is especially important in working with older adults who present with illness, use of multiple medications, and other health concerns.

There are a range of self-administered questionnaires and inventories to supplement the assessment process. The *Handbook of Sexuality-Related Measures* (Davis, Yarber, Bauserman et al., 1998) provides a complete listing and analysis of scales and inventories. While several inventories have been developed specifically for women (e.g., The Female Sexual Function Index; Rosen, Brown, Heiman et al., 2000), there are very few, if any, that are directed primarily toward older adults, and older women in particular (see Malatesta & Adams, 2001).

Sex therapy is a general term for a variously defined group of procedures that include (1) education; (2) communication, intimacy and relationship skill training; and (3) structured behavioral activities. A "mixed model pragmatic approach" is most common. At the same time, there has been a move toward empirically supported treatments to help identify the most effective interventions for sexual dysfunction (see Malatesta & Adams, 2001; Wincze & Carey, 2001).

As health professionals, we obviously must be comfortable, both personally and professionally, with our own sexuality before we can help older adults with their sexual issues. To deal effectively with sexual concerns among older adults, we need to begin with an examination of our own sexual attitudes, beliefs and knowledge regarding sexual behavior. In this regard, there are several organizations that provide education and training for professionals (see Wincze & Carey, 2001, and a listing at the end of the article).

Finally, in working with the sexual needs of older women in particular, any therapeutic intervention should be based upon (1) a solid understanding of the myths and realities of the sexual aging process, (2) a sensitivity to the great variability in sexual beliefs, behaviors and capabilities, (3) a strong endorsement of the broader view of sexuality–one that emphasizes relationship, intimacy and meaning, (4) a keen understanding of the sexual challenges faced by women, (5) a respect for the continuity of one's sexual lifestyle, including sexual activity/inactivity as a nonissue, and (6) a strong willingness to convey an attitude of sexual acceptance, permissiveness and experimentation. In this regard, an important goal is to support the continuity of sexual expression for those whom sexuality has represented an important part of their lives. In other situations, however, it may be as important to validate and support an older client's decision *not* to engage in sexual activity if she so chooses. At the same time, we should be ready to educate, treat, and help find alternative methods of meeting sexual and affectional needs for older women who remain interested in their sexuality but who are disabled, without partners, or living in a restricted environment.

REFERENCES

Anderson, B. L., Woods, X. A., & Copeland, L. J. (1997). Sexual self-schema and sexual morbidity among gynecologic cancer survivors. *Journal of Consulting and Clinical Psychology, 65,* 221-229.

Anllo, L. M. (2000). Sexual life after breast cancer. *Journal of Sex & Marital Therapy, 26,* 241-248.

Basson, R. (2000). The female sexual response: A different model. *Journal of Sex & Marital Therapy, 26,* 51-65.

Basson, R., Leiblum, S., Brotto, L., Derogatis, L., Fourcroy, J., Fugl-Meyer, K. et al. (2003). Definitions of women's sexual dysfunction reconsidered: Advocating expansion and revision. *Journal of Psychosomatic Obstetrics and Gynaecology, 24,* 221-229.

Blank, J. (Ed.) (2000). *Still doing it: Women and men over 60 write about their sexuality.* San Francisco: Down There Press.

Blumberg, E. S. (2003). The lives and voices of highly sexual women. *Journal of Sex Research, 40,* 146-157.

Butler, A. C. (2000). Trends in same-gender sexual partnering, 1988-1998. *Journal of Sex Research, 37,* 333-343.

Cain, V. S., Johannes, C. B., Avis, N. E., Mohr, B. et al. (2003). Sexual functioning and practices in a multi-ethnic study of midlife women: Baseline results from SWAN. *Journal of Sex Research, 40,* 266-276.

Davis, C. M., Yarber, W. L., Bauserman, R., Schreer, G., & Davis, S. L. (1998). *Handbook of sexually-related measures.* Thousand Oaks, CA: Sage.

DeLamater, J. D., & Sill, M. (2005). Sexual desire in later life. *Journal of Sex Research, 42,* 138-149.

Dennerstein, L., Alexander, J. L., & Kotz, K. (2003). The menopause and sexual functioning: A review of the population-based studies. *Annual Review of Sex Research, 14,* 64-82.

Dolan, K. A. (2005). *Lesbian women and sexual health: The social construction of risk and susceptibility.* Binghamton, NY: The Haworth Press, Inc.

Erickson, E. H. (1980). Elements of a psychoanalytic theory of psychosexual development. In S. I. Greenspan & G. H. Pollock (Eds.), *The course of life: Psychoanalytic contributions toward understanding personality development.* Washington, DC: National Institute of Mental Health.

Everaerd, W., & Laan, E. (2000). Drug treatments for women's sexual disorders. *Journal of Sex Research, 37,* 195-204.

George, L. K., & Weiler, S. J. (1981). Sexuality in middle and late life: The effects of age, cohort, and gender. *Archives of Sexual Behavior, 38,* 919-923.

Heiman, J. R. (2002). Sexual dysfunction: Overview of prevalence, etiological factors, and treatments. *Journal of Sex Research, 39,* 73-78.

Hendrick, V., & Gitlin, M. (2004). *Psychotropic drugs and women: Fast facts.* New York: Norton.

Kaplan, H. S. (1974). *The new sex therapy: Active treatment of sexual dysfunctions.* New York: Brunner/Mazel.

Kaplan, H. S. (1979). *Disorders of sexual desire.* New York: Simon & Schuster.

Kaschak, E., & Tiefer, L. (Eds.) (2002). *A new view of women's sexual problems.* Binghamton, NY: The Haworth Press, Inc.

Koch, P. B., Mansfield, P. K., Thurau, D., & Carey, M. (2005). "Feeling frumpy": The relationship between body image and sexual response changes in midlife women. *Journal of Sex Research, 42*, 215-223.

Laumann, E. O., Paik, A., & Rosen, R. C. (1999). Sexual dysfunction in the United States: Prevalence and predictors. *JAMA: Journal of the American Medical Association, 281*, 537-544.

Malatesta, V. J. (1989). Sexuality and the older adult: An Overview with guidelines for The health care professional. *Journal of Women & Aging, 1*, 93-118.

Malatesta, V. J., & Adams, H. E. (2001). Sexual dysfunctions. In H. E. Adams & P. B. Sutker (Eds.), *Comprehensive handbook of psychopathology* (3rd ed., pp. 713-748). New York: Kluwer Academic/Plenum.Human.

Malatesta, V. J., Chambless, D. L., Pollack, M., & Cantor, A. (1988). Widowhood, sexuality and aging: A life span analysis. *Journal of Sex & Marital Therapy, 14*, 49-62.

Malatesta, V. J., Pollack, R. H., Crotty, T. D., & Peacock, L. J. (1982). Acute alcohol intoxication and female orgasmic response. *Journal of Sex Research, 18*, 1-17.

Masters, W. H., & Johnson, V. E. (1966). *Human sexual response.* Boston: Little, Brown.

Masters, W. H., & Johnson, V. E. (1970). *Human sexual inadequacy.* Boston: Little, Brown.

Masters, W. H., Johnson, V. E., & Kolodny, R. C. (1994). *Heterosexuality.* New York: Gramercy.

Meston, C. M., Levin, R. J., Sipski, M. L., Hull, E. M., & Heiman, J. R. (2004). Women's orgasm. *Annual Review of Sex Research, 15*, 173-257.

Michael, R. T., Gagnon, J. H., Laumann, E. O., & Kolata, G. (1994). *Sex in America: A definitive survey.* Boston: Little, Brown.

Montgomery, S. A., Baldwin, D. S., & Riley, A. (2002). Antidepressant medications: A review of the evidence for drug-induced sexual dysfunction. *Journal of Affective Disorders, 69*, 119-140.

Office of the Surgeon General (2001). *The Surgeon General's call to action to promote sexual health and responsible sexual behavior.* Rockville, MD: Office of the Surgeon General.

Rose, S. M. (Ed.) (2002). *Lesbian love and relationships.* Binghamton, NY: The Haworth Press, Inc.

Rosen, R., Brown, C., Heiman, J., Leiblum, S., Meston, C., Shabsigh, R., Ferguson, D., & D'Agostino, Jr., R. (2000). The female sexual function index (FSFI): A multidimensional self-report instrument for the assessment of female sexual function. *Journal of Sex & Marital Therapy, 26*, 191-208.

Sadock, V. A. (1995). Normal human sexuality and sexual and gender identity disorders. In H. I. Kaplan & B. J. Benjamin (Eds.), *Comprehensive textbook of psychiatry* (6th ed., pp. 1295-1321). Baltimore: Williams & Wilkins.

Schover, L. R., & Jensen, S. B. (1988). *Sexuality and chronic illness: A comprehensive Approach.* New York: Guilford.

Siegel, K., & Schrimshaw, E. W. (2003). Reasons for the adoption of celibacy among older men and women living with HIV/AIDS. *Journal of Sex Research, 40*, 189-200.

Tiefer, L. (2001). A new view of women's sexual problems: Why new? Why now? *Journal of Sex Research, 38*, 89-96.

Tiefer, L. (2004). Sex is not a natural act, and other essays (2nd Ed.). Boulder, CO: Westview Press.

Tiggerman, M., & Lynch, J. E. (2002). Body image across the life span in adult women: The role of objectification. *Developmental Psychology, 37*, 243-253.

West, S. L., Vinikoor, L. C., & Zolnoun, D. (2004). A systematic review of the literature on female sexual dysfunction prevalence and predictors. *Annual Review of Sex Research, 15*, 40-172.

Wilsnack, S. C. (1991). Sexuality and women's drinking: Findings from a U. S. national study. *Alcohol Health and Research World, 15*, 147-150.

Wincze, J. P., & Carey, M. P. (2001). *Sexual dysfunction: A guide for assessment and treatment.* New York: Guilford.

For Further Information and Additional Study:

American Association of Sex Educators, Counselors and Therapists: www.aasect.org
International Society for the Study of Women's Sexual Health: www.isswsh.org
Society for Sex Therapy and Research: www.sstarnet.org
Society for the Scientific Study of Sexuality: www.ssc.wisc.edu/ssss/

doi:10.1300/J074v19n01_09

Eating Disorders Across the Life Span

Lynn Brandsma, PhD

SUMMARY. Eating disorders have traditionally been considered af-
flictions of adolescents and young women. Recent evidence, however,
suggests that eating disorders often occur across the life span. Although
the incidence of these disorders among mid-life and older women appears to be on the rise, it is not clear if this reflects a true increase in prevalence, better recognition among clinicians, or both. This paper presents
an overview of the etiology and treatment of eating disorders, with particular emphasis on developmental factors impacting older women. Recommendations for the treatment of eating disorders among older women
are offered. An emerging clinical literature suggests various lines of research that are needed to explore the development and treatment of eating disorders in older women. doi:10.1300/J074v19n01_10 *[Article copies
available for a fee from The Haworth Document Delivery Service: 1-800-
HAWORTH. E-mail address: <docdelivery@haworthpress.com> Website:
<http://www.HaworthPress.com> © 2007 by The Haworth Press, Inc. All rights
reserved.]*

KEYWORDS. Eating disorder, women, aging, bulimia, anorexia, binge
eating

Address correspondence to: Lynn Brandsma, Dept. of Psychology, Chestnut Hill College, 9601 Germantown Ave., Philadelphia, PA 19118 (E-mail: brandsmal@chc.edu).

[Haworth co-indexing entry note]: "Eating Disorders Across the Life Span." Brandsma, Lynn.
Co-published simultaneously in *Journal of Women & Aging* (The Haworth Press, Inc.) Vol. 19, No. 1/2,
2007, pp. 155-172; and: *Mental Health Issues of Older Women: A Comprehensive Review for Health Care
Professionals* (ed: Victor J. Malatesta) The Haworth Press, Inc., 2007, pp. 155-172. Single or multiple copies
of this article are available for a fee from The Haworth Document Delivery Service [1-800-HAWORTH, 9:00
a.m. - 5:00 p.m. (EST). E-mail address: docdelivery@haworthpress.com].

Available online at http://jwa.haworthpress.com
© 2007 by The Haworth Press, Inc. All rights reserved.
doi:10.1300/J074v19n01_10

Eating disorders are broadly defined as any severe and prolonged disturbance in eating behaviors. As a group they are found among 1 to 3% of the population, with more than 90% of the cases occurring in women (American Psychiatric Association, 1994). They are often difficult to treat and remain among the least understood of psychological conditions. Eating disorders have generally been considered disorders of adolescent girls and young women, but emerging evidence has led some to believe that they can occur throughout the life span, and that eating-disordered behavior may in fact be increasing in prevalence among older women. Deep insecurities about one's body image can affect women of all ages, and may set the stage for development of eating disorders in some. This paper will provide an overview of eating disorders and related body image concerns, with a particular emphasis on these disorders through the course of adulthood.

EATING DISORDERS AS DEFINED IN THE DSM-IV

The *Diagnostic and Statistical Manual of Mental Disorders* (DSM-IV; American Psychiatric Association, 1994) classifies eating disorders into three general categories: Anorexia Nervosa (AN), Bulimia Nervosa (BN), and Eating Disorder Not Otherwise Specified (ED-NOS). The latter category includes a variety of conditions in which one meets some, but not all, of the criteria for AN or BN. The principal characteristic of AN is a refusal to maintain body weight at or above a minimally normal standard for age and height. AN is subdivided into Restricting Type or Binge-Eating/Purging Type depending upon whether one only restricts food intake or one also binges and purges but still maintains a body mass index (BMI) below 18. AN can lead to serious health consequences such as heart problems, kidney problems, osteoporosis and bone weakening, and reproductive system damage, among others (Heffner & Eifert, 2004). As many as 20% of AN patients eventually die as a result of the condition, with half of those deaths stemming from suicide (Sullivan, 1995). BN is characterized by recurrent binge eating and inappropriate compensatory behavior such as self-induced vomiting, fasting, or excessive exercise. BN is subdivided into Purging Type (vomiting, or the misuse of laxatives, diuretics, or enemas), which is often confused with AN Binge-Eating/Purging Type, and Nonpurging Type (fasting or excessive exercise). The main distinction between AN binge/purge type and bulimia is body weight (Heffner & Eifert, 2004).

AN is associated with a BMI below 18 whereas the BMI of bulimics is 18 or above (American Psychiatric Association, 1994).

ED-NOS is rarely the focus of research, although patients in this category are quite familiar to practitioners who treat eating disorders (Wilson & Pike, 2001). One of the most prevalent forms of ED-NOS is Binge Eating Disorder (BED). Although BED is technically classified under the ED-NOS umbrella, several scholars have suggested granting it a unique diagnostic status in the future (e.g., Williamson et al., 2002). BED is characterized by recurrent episodes of binge eating that involve eating a large amount of food in a discrete period of time and feeling a lack of control over one's eating during such an episode. Individuals with BED engage in recurrent binge eating, but do not demonstrate the extreme compensatory behavior seen in BN (Wilson & Pike, 2001). They nevertheless resemble patients with BN in many ways, such as dysfunctional concerns with body weight and shape (Wilfley, Schwartz, Spurrell, & Fairburn, 2000), and high rates of comorbid psychopathology, particularly depression (Wilfley, Friedman, Dounchis, Stein, & Welch, 2000). Persons with BED are dissimilar to those with BN in other ways, which have important treatment implications. BED is associated with lower levels of dietary restraint (i.e., utilizing strategies to restrict one's food intake) relative to the other eating disorders (Wilfley, Schwartz et al., 2000). Consequently, the majority of individuals with BED are overweight or obese (Marcus, 1993). More males present with BED than the other eating disorders. Another key difference appears to be that BED affects women in midlife and beyond at a much higher rate than AN or BN.

Phenomenology of Eating Disorders

Each time a media personality goes public with her eating problem a media frenzy tends to follow. Due to a cognitive process known as the availability heuristic (i.e., the tendency to give undue attention to highly vivid or salient information), many assume that eating disorders like AN and BN are extremely common. In fact, when applying the diagnostic criteria outlined in the DSM-IV, the prevalence of AN and BN at any one time is only approximately 0.28% and 1%, respectively (Hoek, 2002). The lifetime prevalence of AN is between 0.5%-1%, and of BN is between 1 and 3% (American Psychiatric Association, 2004). Less epidemiological research has been conducted on BED, but estimates indicate a prevalence of 2 to 3% in the general population and approximately 8% in the obese population (Grilo, 2002).

AN and BN typically have an onset in adolescence (Schwartz & Brownell, 2001). The greatest risk for the development of these eating disorders is during the teenage years and into early adulthood. Although the onset of eating disorders has traditionally been thought to decline thereafter, there is a paucity of good epidemiological data addressing this issue. There have been reports of eating disorders beginning in children as young as seven years of age (Bryant-Waugh & Lask, 2002), as well as one case beginning in a 92-year-old woman (Mermelstein & Basu, 2001). The literature, however, appears mixed about the actual prevalence of those who develop or continue with AN and BN in midlife or beyond. Some scholars suggest that such cases are rare (e.g., Schwartz & Brownell, 2001). However, a growing number of clinicians report that clinical observation and case reports indicate that eating disorders are occurring more frequently in women over 40 (e.g., Kearney-Cooke & Isaacs, 2004). Some suggest that eating disorders tend to be underdiagnosed in midlife and beyond (Hall & Driscoll, 1993; Lewis & Cachelin, 2001). It is likely that eating disorders in women of middle age and beyond are frequently overlooked by health professionals because of the prevailing assumption that eating disorders are only found in adolescent and young women. The data are clearer about the prevalence of BED in older women, suggesting that nearly half of those with BED begin binge eating as an adult (Abbott et al., 1998; Spurrell, Wilfley, Tanofsky, & Brownell, 1997).

Although research on the long-term course of eating disorders is sparse, such data that do exist are somewhat encouraging. A 10-year longitudinal study found that rates of eating disordered behavior dropped by more than half (Heatherton et al., 1997; Vohs, Heatherton, & Herrin, 2001). Such a high rate of remission, however, does not seem to be the case with body image concerns, which are a key concomitant of eating disorders. A study conducted by Lewis and Cachelin (2001) demonstrated that sociocultural standards of body image and pressures toward thinness affect generations of older women in similar ways as younger women. It has only been recently that research on body image and eating disorders has included middle-aged and older women in addition to adolescents and college-aged women. The role of sociocultural factors, including body image dissatisfaction, in the development of eating disorders will be discussed below.

Etiology

There has been considerable theoretical speculation, but surprisingly few solid scientific findings, regarding the etiology of eating disorders.

It is widely believed that certain environmental and personality factors are risk factors for the development of eating disorders (Forman & Davis, 2005). Some of these variables are discussed below.

Psychoanalytic factors. Psychoanalytic theories focus on unresolved unconscious conflicts between the individual and significant others, especially early conflicts with parents. Eating disorders were thought to result from early childhood experiences in which a mother responded to her infant's emotional needs with provision of food or conversely failed to respond to her infant's hunger needs with feeding. Thus, the child never learned to differentiate between physical and emotional needs and also learned to alter her needs to fit those of her caretaker (usually her mother). Subsequently, the eating disordered adolescent strives for autonomy by controlling her intake of food (Bruch, 1978). Such theories dominated the conceptualization and treatment of eating disorders throughout much of the 20th century, but have not been supported by empirical research. Psychoanalytic theories in general have been subjected to increasing criticism over the past few years, and their influence is waning (Crews, 1995; Macmillan, 1997; Cioffi, 1998).

Family factors. Clinicians who treat eating disorders from a family systems perspective have traditionally believed that eating disorders, particularly AN, stem from the individual's efforts to become independent from an overly enmeshed (i.e., involved) family (Minuchin, Rosman, & Baker, 1978). This perspective views disordered eating patterns as a way for the young woman to separate from a family that she sees as blocking her autonomy. In addition to this overcontrolling family style, families that are chaotic, unaffectionate, and insensitive to their child's needs, and those that are incapable of resolving conflict are thought to contribute to the development of eating disorders (Strober & Humphrey, 1987). Little research has evaluated these ideas, and the specificity of these patterns of family conflict and eating disorders, in particular, has not been established. Nevertheless, these ideas continue to be popular among many clinicians, and have led to family interventions being among the more popular psychotherapeutic treatments for eating disorders. Clearly, traditional psychoanalytic and family theories focused solely on adolescent and young women without any mention of eating disorders among middle-aged or older adult women.

Biological factors. Both genetic factors and certain neurotransmitters have been implicated in the etiology of eating disorders. There is considerable evidence that eating disorders are more common among first-degree female relatives of individuals with eating disorders than among women from the population at large (Lilenfeld et al., 1998; Treasure & Holland, 1990). Evidence of familial transmission, however, does not allow discrimination between genetic and environmental influences (Wilson & Pike, 2001). In addition to genetic studies, neurotransmitter function has been a focus of eating disorder research. One neurotransmitter, serotonin, is widely believed to play a part in mood disorders (Keel, Leon, & Fulkerson, 2001). Some patients with eating disorders have responded favorably to antidepressants targeting serotonin, thereby leading to speculation that individuals with eating disorders may also have a serotonin imbalance (Kaye, 2002). Research has indeed found evidence for disturbances in serotonergic neurotransmitter systems in both AN and BN (Kaye, Gwirtsman, George, & Ebert, 1991; Kaye et al., 1998, 2001). However, the research to date does not permit specification of causal pathways. That is, it is not clear whether neurotransmitter disturbances play a role in the cause of the eating disorder or if they are a consequence of eating disorder behavior. Although there is evidence of neurotransmitter disturbances in eating disorders, their causal role, if any, is unclear. It is possible, for example, that neurotransmitter imbalances could reflect the high comorbidity of eating disorders and depression.

Personality factors. Research shows that individuals with eating disorders tend to exhibit perfectionistic traits (Fairburn et al., 1997; Garner & Garfinkel, 1997). It has even been demonstrated that patients who have recovered from AN still score higher on perfectionism than a control group of individuals who have never suffered from an eating disorder (Bastiani, Rao, Weltzin, & Kaye, 1995; Srinivasagam et al., 1995). Women with AN place impossible demands on themselves to obtain the "perfect body" and become frustrated when they cannot achieve it. Bulimic women also tend to be perfectionistic. They tend to engage in dichotomous thinking, seeing the world in stark black and white terms of perfection or failure (Fairburn et al., 1997). This can set the stage for the cycle of bingeing and purging by denying the body food and then bingeing afterwards. Both bulimic and anorexic women are overly concerned about their weight and body shape (Jacobi et al., 2004).

Sociocultural factors. Given the focus on appearance in our society, it is generally accepted that sociocultural factors play more of a role in the etiology of eating disorders than in any other form of psychopathology. It is important to keep in mind, however, that although pressure to conform to the culture's thin ideal is strong, not everyone who is exposed to these pressures develops an eating disorder. Moreover, it is noteworthy that there is evidence to suggest that eating disorders are nearly non-existent in non-Western countries, where the thin body image ideal is not emphasized by the media (Stice, 1994; Wakeling, 1996). In addition, Young, McFatter, and Clopton (2001) demonstrated the role of peer pressure to adhere to a thin body as a strong predictor of bulimic behavior in young women.

Sociocultural norms, as both reflected in and created by the popular media, lead to widespread dissatisfaction with their bodies among many women, and body image dissatisfaction is widely believed to be associated with disordered eating behavior. Body image dissatisfaction is more prevalent in girls than boys (Ricciardelli & McCabe, 2001) and appears to persist across the life span. Girls as young as eight have been known to express dissatisfaction with their bodies (Ricciardelli & McCabe, 2001), as have women as old as 72 (Hsu & Zimmer, 1988). Several studies have shown that middle-aged women appear to be just as preoccupied with their appearance and voice, and many body image concerns, as adolescent and young adult women (Gupta & Schork, 1993; Garner, 1997; Forman & Davis, 2005).

The difficulty developing a healthy body image in adolescence often follows women into and throughout adulthood (Kearney-Cooke & Isaacs, 2004). With thinness being the chief attribute of female beauty, it is no wonder that many American women become obsessed with their bodies and/or develop eating disorders. This obsession that often begins in adolescence continues throughout adulthood. We know that the transition periods from childhood to adolescence and adolescence to young adulthood are associated with increased risk for developing eating disorders and that body image disturbances accompany those disorders (Keel, Leon, & Fulkerson, 2001). Until recently, little attention has been given to the transitions of adulthood with respect to women's views of their bodies.

Adult Developmental Milestones and Eating Disorders

Although most vulnerability factors to psychopathology, including eating disorders, arise before one reaches adulthood, there are certain experiences during the adult years that can trigger the onset of eating problems (Ingram & Fortier, 2001). Certainly, there are many developmental transitions faced by women over 30 that can affect a woman's body image and can precipitate disordered eating.

Zerbe (2003) suggested that the inability to make smooth life transitions or to mourn significant losses such as the death of a loved one, divorce, the "empty nest," and loss of youthfulness can all function as precipitants of eating disorders in middle-aged women. However, since many women struggle with these transitions and only some develop eating disorders, these transitions in and of themselves do not fully address the question of etiology. Nevertheless, it is important to consider such developmental factors in the conceptualization and treatment of eating disorders in older women.

Pregnancy. Differences in eating, weight, and body shape are significant changes for a woman during pregnancy. For some, the postpartum period may leave them vulnerable to the development of an eating disorder (Schwartz & Brownell, 2001). Stein and Fairburn (1996) report that women who retained the most weight after pregnancy were the ones experiencing the most symptoms of an eating disorder. This supports the idea that women may be vulnerable to eating disorder development during the postpartum months. Many women also experience a disturbance in body image during their pregnancy (Schwartz & Brownell, 2001). Rodin (1992) reported that interviews with research subjects and clinical patients suggested that many pregnant women regarded their changed bodies with fear and loathing. The weight gain surrounding pregnancy can be a tremendous source of anxiety and confusion for many women, and the pressure to lose "the baby weight" begins immediately after childbirth. This was not the case 30 or 40 years ago when a woman who had children was expected to be 15 to 20 pounds heavier than before childbirth (Kearney-Cooke & Isaacs, 2004).

Menopause and physical signs of aging. Menopause, generally defined as the cessation of menstruation for 12 consecutive months, usually occurs somewhere between the ages of 41 and 55. The average age of menopause in the United States is currently 51 (Kearney-Cooke & Isaacs, 2004). Although menopause is a natural process, like most transitions, it involves both losses and gains (Kearney-Cooke & Isaacs, 2004). Menopausal symptoms such as hot flashes, mood swings, insomnia, and fatigue can certainly wreak havoc on mind and body. Some have suggested that the physical and emotional changes connected with menopause may be similar to the changes produced by puberty and menarche, resulting in similar eating, weight, and body image concerns in these two different age groups of women (Gupta, 1990; Kellett, Trimble, & Thorley, 1976). Women of menopausal age are increasingly encouraged to stay "fit" and appear youthful, despite the natural signs of aging. Metabolic changes associated with menopause often naturally lead to weight gain. Given the pressures to remain thin, this can prompt an eating disorder type of behavior among some women. In addition, concern over wrinkles and aging skin is often associated with a drive for thinness and excessive dieting. These excessive concerns over natural signs of aging appear to be linked to the development of eating disorders in older women (Gupta, 1995).

Other losses. For many women the role of caretaker for children has been quite constant throughout their adult years. When children leave home and this role is lost, the transition to an "empty nest" can be extremely difficult for some women. According to Kearney-Cooke and Isaacs (2004), some women attempt to cope with this sadness by overeating. Others spend a tremendous amount of energy on diets, face-lifts, and similar attempts to preserve a youthful appearance.

The literature appears mixed about the relationship between marital discord and eating disorders and body image. Some (Abramson, 1999; Dally, 1984) have proposed that marital problems can precipitate disordered eating in older women. Other research (Lewis & Cachelin, 2001) has not found a relationship between marital problems and body image or disordered eating.

Divorce or widowhood may present unique difficulties. Women may suddenly and unexpectedly find themselves single. Among the many challenges this presents, many women experience pressure to look as youthful as possible as they begin to socialize with new friends and even potential dating partners. Again, this may precipitate disordered eating in vulnerable individuals.

TREATMENT

Psychotherapeutic treatments for eating disorders have traditionally focused on the patient's low self-esteem and problems with identity formation. Dysfunctional family patterns and communication style were also typically addressed (Minuchin et al., 1978). However, these treatments were not found to be very effective (Russell, Szmukler, Dare, & Eisler, 1987). More recently, short-term cognitive-behavioral and interpersonal treatments have been developed, which directly address problematic eating behavior and dysfunctional attitudes about body image and weight.

Bulimia Nervosa. Currently, the treatment of choice for BN is cognitive-behavior therapy (CBT) (Wilson & Pike, 2001). The CBT treatment of BN is based on the ground-breaking work of Fairburn (1985). Patients are taught problem-solving techniques (e.g., keeping risky food out of the house), self-control strategies (e.g., self-monitoring), cognitive restructuring (e.g., learning to think differently about body shape and weight as well as eating), and ways to prevent relapse (Fairburn,

1997). It is important to note these CBT strategies represent highly structured interventions, rather than unstructured, informal attempts simply to eat less. Recent research suggests that such informal attempts to restrict eating (known as dietary restraint) are actually associated with poorer outcomes (Wilson & Fairburn, 2002).

It is not uncommon for individuals with BN to be treated with psychotropic medication, most commonly selective serotonergic re-uptake inhibitor antidepressants like fluoxetine (Prozac) (Keel, Leon, & Fulkerson, 2001). Such medications may help to decrease binge frequency and improve mood and preoccupation with weight and shape (Walsh, 2002).

Anorexia Nervosa. Psychopharmacologic treatments have not been found to be as effective in the treatment of AN (Attia, Haiman, Walsh, & Flater, 1998; Garner & Needleman, 1996; Vitiello & Lederhendler, 2000). Although therapies for BN have been based on controlled studies that provide a basis for informed judgment about the efficacy of treatment (e.g., Fairburn et al., 1993, 1995; Walsh & Garner, 1997; Wilson & Fairburn, 1993, 2002), this is not the case for the treatment of AN. It is well-established that weight gain is the first goal of treatment for individuals with AN due to the serious medical complications associated with dangerously low weight. Because anorexic patients share similar features to those with bulimia, CBT is often employed. Although data are limited, it appears that CBT approaches that target distorted beliefs about weight and food, as well as those about the self, are more effective than nutritional counseling or drug therapy alone (Vitousek, 2002).

One promising approach is a variation of CBT that integrates mindfulness and acceptance strategies. Rather than focusing on changing the content of negative cognitions, these approaches foster detachment from and acceptance of distressing experiences (e.g., thoughts, beliefs, sensations) in the context of specific behavior change efforts. There has recently been a dramatic increase in interest in such treatments, and initial data are promising (Hayes, Luoma, Bond, Masuda, & Lillis, in press). Among the best established of these new approaches is Acceptance and Commitment Therapy (ACT; Hayes & Strosahl, 2005; Hayes, Strosahl, & Wilson, 1999). An ACT-based protocol for AN was recently published (Heffner & Eifert, 2004), as was a case report based on the successful treatment of a young woman with AN (Heffner, Sperry, Eifert, & Detweiler, 2002).

Binge Eating Disorder. Due to the relatively recent recognition of BED, few empirical studies have been conducted on its treatment. Results by Smith, Marcus, and Kaye (1992), in which CBT treatments for

BN were adapted to obese binge eaters, appear promising. The focus of their treatment as well as that conducted by Agras, Telch, Arnow, Eldredge, and Marnell (1997) has been on stopping binge eating. Cessation of binge eating in obese patients appears to be a consistent, critical component of weight-loss procedures (Marcus, Wing, & Hopkins, 1988; Telch, Agras, & Rossiter, 1988).

There has been considerable controversy regarding the potential role of dieting in promoting binge eating and long-term weight gain. Polivy and Herman (1993) theorized that dietary restraint (i.e., the tendency to utilize cognitive strategies to restrict one's food intake) is associated with increased binge frequency. Indeed, several studies have supported such a relationship (e.g., Wilfley, Pike, & Striegel-Moore, 1997). This has led to a question concerning the use of diets, especially among those with a history of binge eating. Lowe (1993) argued that dietary restraint as operationalized by the Restraint Scale (Herman & Polivy, 1980) in these studies is different from current dieting to lose weight. Dietary restraint refers to chronic but unstructured attempts to maintain a negative energy balance which, not surprisingly, often leads to struggles with food, binge eating, and eventual weight gain. In contrast, explicit dieting has been shown to result not only in weight loss, but in decreased binge frequency as well, even in at risk populations (National Task Force on the Prevention and Treatment of Obesity, 2000). This research highlights the importance of highly structured eating plans in individuals with BED.

Guidelines for Clinicians for Working with Adult Women

Given the widespread stereotype of eating disorders as problems of adolescents and young women, it is critical that clinicians be aware of the possibility of eating disorders across the life span. Although hard data are lacking, it appears increasingly likely that the prevalence of eating disorders, both in terms of new onset as well as unremitted cases, is increasing among middle-aged and older women. The first step to appropriate treatment is recognition.

The present review did not reveal any controlled outcome trials of interventions for eating disorders specifically targeting older adult women. This suggests that the most prudent course of action is to utilize empirically supported treatments that have been developed and evaluated with younger women, with appropriate modifications for working with older adults.

One advantage of working with older individuals is that one can explore coping strategies that have and have not worked in the past. Older women have more history from which to glean both potentially useful coping strategies as well as those that are unlikely to be helpful. Although many of the issues facing middle-aged and older women are markedly different than those of adolescent and young women, cognitive restructuring related to body image concerns would still be appropriate. The difference is that in middle-aged and older women these concerns are typically examined in the context of fears regarding aging.

Education about realistic weight expectations is also likely to be helpful. Body fat increases and metabolism decreases with age. Many women have borne children, which often results in permanent changes in body shape. Changing estrogen levels during menopause may cause body fat to redistribute in the waist and stomach. All of these changes make weight loss more difficult (Kearney-Cooke & Isaacs, 2004). People tend to look heavier as they age, even if their weight does not change, and this effect is especially true for older women (Williamson, Kahn, & Remington, 1990). Women are often forced with a choice between expending large amounts of time and energy attempting to become or stay unrealistically thin or accepting being a few pounds heavier than in their younger years.

It also needs to be recognized that obesity is an increasing health concern in North America. Clinicians must reconcile the client's binge eating and cognitive distortions regarding the thin ideal with the reality of the growing epidemic of obesity. Professionals need to be sensitive to the data on the pernicious effects of dietary restraint, yet be cautious about undermining efforts at appropriate weight control. Lowe and Timko (2004) reviewed data suggesting that dieting behavior may be harmful, ineffective, or actually helpful, both in terms of weight control and eating disorder symptoms, depending upon a variety of contextual factors. Blanket prohibitions against dieting are overly simplistic; current evidence calls for a more nuanced approach.

FUTURE DIRECTIONS

Epidemiological research is needed to identify the prevalence of eating disorders in middle-aged and older adult women. It is important to know if this apparent increase in cases reflects a greater recognition among clinicians, an actual increase in prevalence, or perhaps both. Such research can set the stage for exploring additional issues that may have both etiological and treatment implications (e.g., whether late on-set eating disorders differ from those that begin earlier in life).

There is an urgent need for treatment development efforts focused specifically on middle-aged and older adult women. Evaluating medications specifically for eating-disordered behavior for this particular age group of women is necessary. In addition, variations of cognitive behavioral therapy, including the newer acceptance-based models such as ACT, need to be developed and evaluated. All psychotherapeutic approaches utilized should be sensitive to the developmental factors associated with this population.

Finally, educational efforts among health-care professionals, especially primary care physicians, gynecologists, mental health professionals, and others who regularly work with women regarding appropriate recognition and diagnosis of eating disorders in middle-aged and older adult women, is essential. Treatment cannot take place unless one first recognizes the problem.

REFERENCES

Abbott, D.W., deZwann, M., Mussell, M.P., Raymond, N.C., Seim, H.C., Crow, S.J., Crosby, R.D., & Mitchell, J.E. (1998). Onset of binge eating and dieting in over-weight women: Implications for etiology, associated features and treatment. *Journal of Psychosomatic Research, 44,* 367-374.

Abramson, E.E. (1999). *To have and to hold: How to take off the weight when marriage puts on the pounds.* New York: Kensington Books.

Agras, W.S., Telch, C.F., Arnow, B., Eldredge, K., & Marnell, M. (1997). One year follow-up of cognitive-behavioral therapy of obese individuals with binge eating disorder. *Journal of Consulting and Clinical Psychology, 65,* 343-347.

American Psychiatric Association (1994). *Diagnostic and statistical manual of mental disorders* (4th ed.). Washington, DC: Author.

Attia, E., Haiman, C., Walsh, B.T., & Flater, S.R. (1998). Does fluoxetine augment the inpatient treatment of anorexia nervosa? *American Journal of Psychiatry, 155(4),* 548-551.

Bastiani, A.M., Rao, R., Weltzin, T., & Kaye, W.H. (1995). Perfectionism in anorexia nervosa. *International Journal of Eating Disorders, 17(2),* 147-152.

Bruch, H. (1978). *The golden cage.* New York: Vintage Books.

Bryant-Waugh, R., & Lask, B. (2002). Childhood-onset eating disorders. In C.G. Fairburn & K.D. Brownell (Eds.), *Eating disorders and obesity: A comprehensive handbook* (2nd ed.; pp. 210-214). New York: Guilford Press.

Cioffi, F. (1998). *Freud and the question of pseudoscience.* Peru, IL: Carus.

Crews, F. (1995). *The memory wars: Freud's legacy in dispute.* New York: The New York Review of Books.

Dally, P. (1984). Anorexia tardive-late onset marital anorexia nervosa. *Journal of Psychosomatic Research, 28*, 423-428.

Fairburn, C.G. (1985). Cognitive-behavioral treatment for bulimia. In D.M. Clark Garner & P.E. Garfinkel (Eds.), *Handbook of psychotherapy for anorexia nervosa and bulimia* (pp. 160-192). New York: Guilford Press.

Fairburn, C.G. (1997). Eating disorders. In D.M. Clark & C.G. Fairburn (Eds.), *The science and practice of cognitive behaviour therapy*. Oxford, U.K.: Oxford University Press.

Fairburn, C.G., Jones, R., Peveler, R.C., Hope, R.A., & O'Connor, M. (1993). Psychotherapy and bulimia nervosa: Long-term effects of interpersonal psychotherapy, behavior therapy, and cognitive behavior therapy. *Archives of General Psychiatry, 50(6)*, 419-428.

Fairburn, C.G., Norman, P.A., Welch, S.L., O'Connor, M.E., Doll, H.A., & Peveler, R.C. (1995). A prospective outcome of bulimia nervosa and the long-term effects of three psychological treatments. *Archives of General Psychiatry, 52(4)*, 304-312.

Fairburn, C.G., Welch, S.L., Doll, H.A., Davies, B.A., & O'Connor, M.E. (1997). Risk factors for bulimia nervosa: A community-based case-control study. *Archives of General Psychiatry, 54(6)*, 509-517.

Forman, M., & Davis, W.N. (2005). Characteristics of middle-aged women in inpatient treatment for eating disorders. *Eating Disorders: The Journal of Treatment and Prevention, 13*, 231-243.

Garner, D.M. (1997). The 1997 body image results. *Psychology Today*.

Garner, D.M., & Garfinkel, P.E. (Eds.) (1997). *Handbook of treatment for eating disorders* (2nd ed.). New York: Guilford Press.

Garner, D.M., & Needleman, L.D. (1996). Step care and the decision-tree models for treating eating disorders. In J.K. Thompson (Ed.), *Body image, eating disorders and obesity* (pp. 225-252). Washington, DC: American Psychological Association.

Grilo, C.M. (2002). Binge eating disorder. In C.G. Fairburn & K.D. Brownell (Eds.), *Eating disorders and obesity: A comprehensive handbook* (2nd ed.; pp. 178-182). New York: Guilford Press.

Gupta, M.A. (1990). Fear of aging: A precipitating factor in late onset anorexia nervosa. *International Journal of Eating Disorders, 2*, 15-34.

Gupta, M.A. (1995). Concerns about aging and a drive for thinness: A factor in the biopsychosocial model of eating disorders? *International Journal of Eating Disorders, 18*, 351-357.

Gupta, M.A., & Schork, N. (1993). Aging-related concerns and body image: Possible future implications for eating disorders. *International Journal of Eating Disorders, 14*, 481-486.

Hall, P., & Driscoll, R. (1993). Anorexia in the elderly–an annotation. *International Journal of Eating Disorders, 14*, 497-499.

Hayes, S.C., Luoma, J.B., Bond, F.W., Masuda, A., & Lillis, J. (in press). Acceptance and Commitment Therapy: Model, processes and outcomes. *Behaviour Research and Therapy*.

Hayes, S.C. & Strosahl, K.D. (2005) (Eds.). *A practical guide to Acceptance and Commitment Therapy*. New York: Springer-Verlag.

Hayes, S.C., Strosahl, K., & Wilson, K.G. (1999). *Acceptance and Commitment Therapy: An experiential approach to behavior change.* New York: Guilford Press.

Heatherton, T.F., Mahamedi, F., Striepe, M., Field, A.E., & Keel, P. (1997). A 10-year longitudinal study of body weight, dieting, and eating disorder symptoms. *Journal of Abnormal Psychology, 106,* 117-125.

Heffner, M., & Eifert, G.H. (2004). *The Anorexia workbook: How to accept yourself, heal your suffering, and reclaim your life.* Oakland CA: New Harbinger.

Heffner, M., Sperry, J., Eifert, G.H. & Detweiler, M. (2002). Acceptance and Commitment Therapy in the treatment of an adolescent female with anorexia nervosa: A case example. *Cognitive and Behavioral Practice, 9,* 232-236.

Herman, C.P., & Polivy, J. (1980). Restrained eating. In A.J. Stunkard (Ed.), *Obesity* (pp. 208-225). Philadelphia: Saunders.

Hoek, H.W. (2002). Distribution of eating disorders. In C.G. Fairburn & K.D. Brownell (Eds.), *Eating disorders and obesity: A comprehensive handbook* (2nd ed.; pp. 233-237). New York: Guilford Press.

Hsu, L.K.G., & Zimmer, B. (1988). Eating disorders in old age. *International Journal of Eating Disorders, 7(1),* 133-138.

Ingram, R.E., & Fortier, M. (2001). The nature of adult vulnerability: History and definitions. In R.E. Ingram & J.M. Price (Eds.), *Vulnerability to psychopathology: Risk across the lifespan* (pp. 39-54). New York: Guilford Press.

Jacobi, C., Hayward, C., deZwaan, M., Kraemer, H.C., & Agras, W.S. (2004). Coming to terms with risk factors for eating disorders: Application of risk terminology and suggestions for a general taxonomy. *Psychological Bulletin, 130,* 19-65.

Kaye, W.H. (2002). Central nervous system neurotransmitter activity in anorexia nervosa and bulimia nervosa. In C.G. Fairburn & K.D. Brownell (Eds.), *Eating disorders and obesity: A comprehensive handbook* (2nd ed.; pp. 272-277). New York: Guilford Press.

Kaye, W.H., Frank, G.K., Meltzer, C.C., Price, J.C., McConaha, C.W., Crossan, P.J., Klump, K.L., & Rhodes, L. (2001). Altered serotonin 2A receptor activity in women who have recovered from bulimia nervosa. *American Journal of Psychiatry, 158(7),* 1152-1155.

Kaye, W.H., Greeno, C.G., Moss, H., Fernstrom, J., Fernstrom, M., Lilenfeld, L.R., Weltzin, T.E., & Mann, J.J. (1998). Alterations in serotonin activity and psychiatric symptoms after recovery from bulimia nervosa. *Archives of General Psychiatry, 55,* 927-935.

Kaye, W.H., Gwirtsman, H.E., George, D.T., & Ebert, M.H. (1991). Altered serotonin activity in anorexia nervosa after long-term weight restoration. *Archives of General Psychiatry, 48,* 556-562.

Kearney-Cooke, A., & Isaacs, F. (2004). *Change your mind, change your body: Feeling good about your body and self after 40.* New York: Atria.

Keel, P.K., Leon, G.R., & Fulkerson, J.A. (2001). Vulnerability to eating disorders in childhood and adolescence. In R.E. Ingram & J.M. Price (Eds.), *Vulnerability to psychopathology: Risk across the lifespan* (pp. 389-411). New York: Guilford Press.

Kellett, J., Trimble, M., & Thorley, A. (1976). Anorexia nervosa after the menopause. *British Journal of Psychiatry, 128,* 555-558.

Lewis, D., & Cachelin, F. (2001). Body image, body dissatisfaction, and eating attitudes in midlife and elderly women. *Eating Disorders: The Journal of Treatment and Prevention, 9,* 29-39.

Lilenfeld, L.R., Kaye, W.H., Greeno, C.G., Merikangas, K.R., Plotnicov, K., Pollice, C., Rao, R., Strober, M., Bulik, C.M., & Nagy, L. (1998). A controlled family study of anorexia nervosa and bulimia nervosa: Psychiatric disorders in first-degree relatives and effects of proband comorbidity. *Archives of General Psychiatry, 55,* 603-610.

Lowe, M.R. (1993). The effects of dieting on eating behavior: A three-factor model. *Psychological Bulletin, 114,* 100-121.

Lowe, M.R., & Timko, C.A. (2004). Dieting: really harmful, merely ineffective or actually helpful? *British Journal of Nutrition, 92,* S19-S22.

Macmillan, M. (1997). *Freud evaluated: The completed arc.* Cambridge, MA: MIT Press.

Marcus, M.D. (1993). Binge eating in obesity. In C.G. Fairburn & G.T. Wilson (Eds.), *Binge eating: Nature, assessment and treatment* (pp. 77-96). New York: Guilford Press.

Marcus, M.D., Wing, R.R., & Hopkins, J. (1988). Obese binge eaters: Affect, cognitions, and response to behavioral weight control. *Journal of Consulting and Clinical Psychology, 3,* 433-439.

Mermelstein, H.T., & Basu, R. (2001). Can you ever be too old or too thin? Anorexia nervosa in a 92-year-old woman. *International Journal of Eating Disorders, 30(1),* 123-126.

Minuchin, S., Rosman, B.L., & Baker, L. (1978). *Psychosomatic families: Anorexia nervosa in context.* Cambridge, MA: Harvard University Press.

National Task Force on the Prevention and Treatment of Obesity (2000). Dieting and the development of eating disorders in overweight and obese adults. *Archives of Internal Medicine, 160,* 2581-2589.

Polivy, J., & Herman, C.P. (1993). Etiology of binge eating: Psychological mechanisms. In C.G. Fairburn & G.T. Wilson (Eds.), *Binge eating: Nature, assessment, and treatment* (pp. 173-205). New York: Guilford Press.

Ricciardelli, L.A., & McCabe, M.P. (2001). Children's body image concerns and eating disturbance: A review of the literature. *Clinical Psychology Review, 21,* 325-344.

Rodin, J. (1992). *Body traps.* New York: William Morrow.

Russell, G.F.M., Szmukler, G.I., Dare, C., & Eisler, I. (1987). An evaluation of family therapy in anorexia nervosa and bulimia nervosa. *Archives of General Psychiatry, 44,* 1047-1056.

Schwartz, M.B., & Brownell, K.D. (2001). Vulnerability to eating disorders in adulthood. In R.E. Ingram & J.M. Price (Eds.), *Vulnerability to psychopathology: Risk across the lifespan* (pp. 412-446). New York: Guilford Press.

Smith, D.E., Marcus, M.D., & Kaye, W. (1992). Cognitive-behavioral treatment of obese binge eaters. *International Journal of Eating Disorders, 12,* 257-262.

Spurrell, E.B., Wilfley, D.E., Tanofsky, M.C., & Brownell, K.D. (1997). Age of onset for binge eating: Are there different pathways to binge eating? *International Journal of Eating Disorders, 21,* 55-65.

Srinivasagam, N.M., Kaye, W.H., Plotnicov, K.H., Greeno, C., Weltzin, T.E., & Rao, R. (1995). Persistent perfectionism, symmetry, and exactness after long-term recovery from anorexia nervosa. *American Journal of Psychiatry, 152,* 1630-1634.

Stein, A., & Fairburn, C.G. (1996). Eating habits and attitudes in the postpartum period. *Psychosomatic Medicine, 58,* 321-325.

Stice, E. (1994). Review of the evidence for a sociocultural model of bulimia nervosa and an exploration of the mechanisms of action. *Clinical Psychology Review, 14,* 633-661.

Strober, M., & Humphrey, L.L. (1987). Familial contributions to the etiology and course of anorexia nervosa and bulimia. *Journal of Consulting and Clinical Psychology, 55,* 654-659.

Sullivan, P.F. (1995). Mortality in anorexia nervosa. *American Journal of Psychiatry 152,* 1073-1074.

Telch, C.F., Agras, W.S., & Rossiter, E.M. (1988). Binge eating increases with increasing adiposity. *International Journal of Eating Disorders, 7,* 115-119.

Treasure, J., & Holland, A. (1990). Genetic vulnerability to eating disorders: Evidence from twin and family studies. In H. Remschmidt & M.H. Schmidt (Eds.), *Child and youth psychiatry: European perspectives* (pp. 59-68). Lewiston, NY: Hogrefe & Huber.

Vitiello, B., & Lederhendler, I. (2000). Research on eating disorders: Current status and future prospects. *Biological Psychiatry, 47,* 777-786.

Vitousek, K.B. (2002). Cognitive-behavioral therapy for anorexia nervosa. In C.G. Fairburn & K.D. Brownell (Eds.), *Eating disorders and obesity: A comprehensive handbook* (2nd ed.; pp. 308-313). New York: Guilford Press.

Vohs, K.D., Heatherton, T.F., & Herrin, M. (2001). Disordered eating and the transition to college: A prospective study. *International Journal of Eating Disorders, 29,* 280-288.

Wakeling, A. (1996). Epidemiology of anorexia nervosa. *Psychiatry Research, 62,* 3-9.

Walsh, B.T. (2002). Pharmacological treatment of anorexia nervosa and bulimia nervosa. In C.G. Fairburn & K.D. Brownell (Eds.), *Eating disorders and obesity: A comprehensive handbook* (2nd ed.; pp. 325-329). New York: Guilford Press.

Walsh, B.T., & Garner, D.M. (1997). Diagnostic issues. In D.M. Garner & P.E. Garfinkel (Eds.), *Handbook of treatment for eating disorders* (pp. 25-33). New York: Guilford Press.

Wilfley, D.E., Friedman, M.A., Dounchis, J.Z., Stein, R.I., & Welch, R. (2000). Comorbid psychopathology in binge eating disorder: Relation to eating disorder severity at baseline and following treatment. *Journal of Consulting and Clinical Psychology, 68,* 295-305.

Wilfley, D.E., Pike, K.M., & Striegel-Moore, R.H. (1997). Toward an integrated model of risk for binge eating disorder. *Journal of Gender, Culture, and Health, 2,* 1-32.

Wilfley, D.E., Schwartz, M.N.B., Spurrell, E.B., & Fairburn, C.G. (2000). Using the Eating Disorder Examination to identify the specific psychopathology of binge eating disorder. *International Journal of Eating Disorders, 27,* 259-269.

Williamson, D.A., Womble, L.G., Smeets, M.A.M., Netemeyer, R.G., Thaw, J.M., Kutlesic, V., & Gleaves, D.H. (2002). Latent structure of eating disorder symptoms: A factor analytic and taxometric investigation. *American Journal of Psychiatry, 159*, 412-418.

Williamson, D.F., Kahn, H.S., & Remington, P.L. (1990). The ten-year incidence of overweight and major weight gain in U.S. adults. *Archives of Internal Medicine, 150*, 665-672.

Wilson, G.T., & Fairburn, C.G. (1993). Cognitive treatments for eating disorders. *Journal of Consulting and Clinical Psychology, 61*, 261-269.

Wilson, G.T., & Fairburn, C.G. (2002). Treatments for eating disorders. In P.E. Nathan & J.M. Gorman (Eds.), *A guide to treatments that work* (2nd ed.; pp. 559-592). New York: Oxford University Press.

Wilson, G.T., & Pike, K.M. (2001). Eating disorders. In D.H. Barlow (Ed.), *Clinical handbook of psychological disorders* (3rd ed.; pp. 332-375). New York: Guilford Press.

Young, E.A., McFatter, R., & Clopton, J.R. (2001). Family functioning, peer influence, and media influence as predictors of bulimic behavior. *Eating Behaviors, 2*, 323-337.

Zerbe, K.J. (2003). Eating disorders in middle and late life: A neglected problem. *Primary Psychiatry, 10*, 80-82.

doi:10.1300/J074v19n01_10

Borderline Personality Disorder Across the Life Span

Melissa Hunt, PhD

SUMMARY. Borderline personality disorder is characterized by affective dysregulation, intense, unstable interpersonal relationships, impulsivity and unstable identity. It overlaps considerably with both PTSD and bipolar spectrum disorders. Research on true late-life BPD is limited, but suggests that some of the core features of BPD including interpersonal difficulties, unstable affect and anger remain relatively unchanged, while impulsivity and identity disturbance decline or change their mode of expression in late life. Diagnosis of BPD in late life requires flexible application of the standard diagnostic criteria as well as a thorough longitudinal history. The etiology of BPD is best explained as a combination of genetic, neurobiological vulnerability combined with childhood trauma, abuse or neglect that leads to dysregulated emotions, distorted cognitions, social skills deficits, and few adaptive coping strategies. Treatment options include pharmacotherapy (especially mood stabilizers, SSRIs and atypical antipsychotics) and psychotherapeutic interventions that focus on distress tolerance, affective regulation, changing distorted beliefs, and introducing new social and relationship problem-solving skills (especially Dialectical Behavior Therapy and Schema Focused Cognitive Therapy). In late-life care environments,

---

Address correspondence to: Melissa Hunt, Dept. of Psychology, University of Pennsylvania, 3720 Walnut St., Philadelphia, PA 19104-6241 (E-mail: Mhunt@psych.upenn.edu).

[Haworth co-indexing entry note]: "Borderline Personality Disorder Across the Life Span." Hunt, Melissa. Co-published simultaneously in *Journal of Women & Aging* (The Haworth Press, Inc.) Vol. 19, No. 1/2, 2007, pp. 173-191; and: *Mental Health Issues of Older Women: A Comprehensive Review for Health Care Professionals* (ed: Victor J. Malatesta) The Haworth Press, Inc., 2007, pp. 173-191. Single or multiple copies of this article are available for a fee from The Haworth Document Delivery Service [1-800-HAWORTH, 9:00 a.m. - 5:00 p.m. (EST). E-mail address: docdelivery@haworthpress.com].

such as nursing homes and other residential facilities, staff need to be empowered to set appropriate limits on problematic behavior while maintaining empathy and validating the painful affect patients often experience. doi:10.1300/J074v19n01_11 *[Article copies available for a fee from The Haworth Document Delivery Service: 1-800-HAWORTH. E-mail address: <docdelivery@haworthpress.com> Website: <http://www.HaworthPress.com> © 2007 by The Haworth Press, Inc. All rights reserved.]*

KEYWORDS. Borderline, personality disorder, women, aging, character

INTRODUCTION

Borderline personality disorder is the quintessential personality disorder. Starting in adolescence and continuing more or less unchanged at least until the early to mid-40s, its hallmark symptoms include intense and highly unstable affect, intense and highly unstable relationships, poor impulse control, and an overwhelming, painful sense of emptiness. Some patients with BPD engage in self-mutilatory or other non-fatal self-harming behaviors. Some make frequent suicide attempts. Indeed, the 10 to 15 year mortality rate (secondary to suicide) for individuals with BPD is approximately 10% (Paris, 2002). There is considerable debate about the course of BPD in later life, with most research suggesting that while many of the core features of BPD persist into late life, there are also significant changes in the presentation of the disorder (Rosowsky & Gurian, 1991; Trappler & Backfield, 2001).

Prevalence

Epidemiological data suggest that the prevalence of BPD in the general community is approximately 1.8% (Swartz, Blazer, George & Winfield, 1990). Widiger and Weissman (1991) in a comprehensive review reported that various studies have estimated a prevalence range from .2 to 2.8%. They also noted that rates of BPD are significantly higher among psychiatric inpatients (15%), while BPD cases comprise 50% of personality disorders among psychiatric inpatients. There is a considerable sex difference, with women outnumbering men three to one.

DIAGNOSTIC CRITERIA

The gold standard in diagnostic criteria for mental disorders is the DSM-IV, the Diagnostic and Statistical Manual for Mental Disorders, 4th

Edition (American Psychiatric Association, 1994). The specific criteria for BPD are as follows: BPD is characterized in the DSM-IV as "a pervasive pattern of instability of interpersonal relationships, self-image, and affects, and marked impulsivity beginning by early adulthood and present in a variety of contexts, as indicated by five (or more) of the following:

1. Frantic efforts to avoid real or imagined abandonment (not including suicidal or self-mutilating behavior).
2. A pattern of unstable and intense interpersonal relationships characterized by alternating between extremes of idealization and devaluation.
3. Identity disturbance: markedly and persistently unstable self-image or sense of self.
4. Impulsivity in at least two areas that are potentially self-damaging (e.g., spending, sex, substance abuse, reckless driving, binge eating) (but not including suicidal or self-mutilating behavior).
5. Recurrent suicidal behavior, gestures, threats or self-mutilating behavior.
6. Affective instability due to a marked reactivity of mood (e.g., intense episodic dysphoria, irritability, or anxiety usually lasting a few hours and only rarely more than a few days).
7. Chronic feelings of emptiness.
8. Inappropriate, intense anger or difficulty controlling anger (e.g., frequent displays of temper, constant anger, recurrent physical fights).
9. Transient, stress-related paranoid ideation or severe dissociative symptoms" (p. 654).

The most widely-used structured diagnostic interview for BPD is the Revised Diagnostic Interview for Borderlines (DIB-R) (Zanarini, Gunderson, Frankenburg & Chauncey, 1989). The DIB-R distinguishes four main categories of symptoms including interpersonal difficulties, affective disturbance, cognitive disturbance and impulsivity.

DIFFERENTIAL DIAGNOSIS AND COMORBIDITY

Interestingly, the features of BPD overlap considerably with both PTSD and Bipolar spectrum disorders. Not surprisingly, there are high comorbidity rates between BPD and these disorders, and differential diagnosis can sometimes be difficult.

PTSD. PTSD has several core features that overlap with BPD, including affective instability (particularly anger/irritability), numb or empty feelings and interpersonal dysfunction (Zlotnick, Johnson, Yen et al., 2003). Moreover, there is considerable comorbidity between the two diagnoses. Zanarini, Frankenburg, Dubo et al. (1998) found comorbid PTSD in 56% of a sample of patients with BPD. At the same time, Shea, Zlotnick and Weisberg (1999) found that 68% of PTSD patients they examined also met diagnostic criteria for BPD.

This has led to considerable debate about the conceptual differences between PTSD and BPD (see Gunderson & Sabo, 1993a; Kudler, 1993; Gunderson & Sabo, 1993b). Gunderson and Sabo (1993a) point out that many BPD patients experienced significant trauma in their early lives and are therefore quite vulnerable to developing PTSD. They point out the enduring effects that trauma (especially early trauma) can have on the formation of personality traits. Zlotnick, Johnson, Yen et al. (2003) examined the clinical features, level of impairment and trauma histories of women with BPD versus women with both BPD and PTSD. They found that co-morbid PTSD increased both hospitalizations and general dysfunction. They found that most of their subjects (89%) had experienced some type of abuse from a primary caretaker before the age of 13. For the comorbid BPD and PTSD group, there were higher rates of sexual, physical, verbal and emotional abuse than in the BPD alone group. The important point to keep in mind for those working clinically with BPD is that trauma history is often highly relevant, and that it can be helpful both to the clinician and the patient to conceptualize certain aspects of BPD as related to trauma survival and chronic PTSD.

Affective and Bipolar Spectrum Disorders. There is also considerable overlap between the core features of BPD and a number of affective disorders, including major depressive disorder, atypical depression, bipolar disorder, and various bipolar spectrum disorders including bipolar II and cyclothymia. Akiskal (1985) was one of the first to point out that the affective symptoms of BPD were central features and probably represented a core temperamental vulnerability. He and his colleagues also suggested that BPD could best be conceptualized as falling within the broad spectrum of bipolar disorders (Akiskal, 1981; Akiskal, Hirschfield, & Yerevanian, 1983).

These similarities can make differential diagnosis difficult. Smith, Muir and Blackwood (2005) examined 87 patients who met criteria for bipolar disorder, bipolar spectrum disorder or major depressive disorder. While none of the patients in the study met diagnostic criteria for

BPD, patients with bipolar disorder endorsed significantly higher numbers of borderline symptoms than did patients with unipolar depression.

Bellino, Patria, Paradiso et al. (2005) found that severity of BPD pathology in depressed individuals was positively correlated with the occurrence of mood disorders in first-degree relatives. They concluded that patients with co-morbid MDD and BPD showed a stronger familial link with mood disorders than is shown by depressed patients with other Axis II disorders, strongly suggesting that BPD may share at least some of the genetic basis of mood disorders.

Moreover, there is considerable overlap between BPD and atypical depression. Atypical depression is defined by mood reactivity, rejection sensitivity, increased appetite and hypersomnia. Many people diagnosed with atypical depression go on to experience an episode of hypomania and are ultimately diagnosed with bipolar II (Akiskal, Walker, Puzantian et al., 1983; Perugi, Akiskal, Lattanzi et al., 1998). Perugi, Toni, Travierso and Akiskal (2003) found that this same cluster of atypical symptoms was common among depressed borderline patients. Perugi and Akiskal (2002) argued persuasively that BPD belongs within a broad clinical group that includes atypical depression and bipolar disorder, and that all three stem, in part, from an underlying cyclothymic temperament, or biological affective lability. Smith, Muir and Blackwood (2004) reviewed recent work in neurobiology on the phenomenology of these disorders, and on the efficacy of mood stabilizers in the management of BPD symptoms, and strongly supported the utility of conceptualizing BPD as a bipolar spectrum disorder. They point out that "since borderline patients can be so challenging to care for, it may be that a reframing of the disorder as belonging to the broad clinical spectrum of bipolar disorders holds benefits for patients and clinicians alike" (page 133).

On the other hand, it is also important to note that BPD remains a separate disorder that imposes unique burdens on the patient, and unique challenges to the clinician. Thinking of it as a bipolar spectrum disorder is therapeutically useful, but does not address the significant skills deficits, the trauma history, the unstable interpersonal relationships or the intensity of continual crisis management that is often required early in treatment. McGill (2004), while acknowledging the considerable evidence in favor of classing BPD with the bipolar disorders, cautioned that BPD itself is still a valid diagnosis, and that careful consideration of the patient's longitudinal history is crucial to establishing the correct diagnosis.

DIAGNOSIS IN LATE LIFE

There is a striking lack of relevant research on BPD in true late life, with most studies examining patients in their 40s and 50s. For example, in one study of older patients with BPD, the oldest patient was only 52 (Stevenson, Meares & Comerford, 2003). Nevertheless, some conclusions can be drawn about the course of BPD into later life. In one widely cited study, Reich, Nduaguba and Yates (1988) found that the trajectory of Cluster B personality disorder traits followed a reverse J shaped curve, with the mean number of traits declining as subjects aged into their 40s and 50s, but then increasing again slightly as subjects aged past 60.

Other authors have noted that there is a change in the pattern of symptoms as BPD patients age. In particular, they appear to become less impulsive over time, although it may be that behavioral expression of impulsivity simply changes. Stevenson, Meares and Comerford (2003) found that age significantly predicted declines in the impulsivity category on the DIB-R, but did not predict declines in affective or relationship disturbance. There was a trend toward reduction in cognitive disturbance as well, but it was not significant using their stringent criteria.

Paris and Zweig-Frank (2001) conducted a 27-year follow-up of a cohort of BPD patients they had originally assessed in the 1980s. The mean age of their sample was 51. In contrast to the above study, they found that there were no significant changes in impulsivity, while there were large and highly significant decreases in relationship difficulties. Their most striking finding was that only 8% of patients continued to meet criteria for BPD using the DIB-R. They interpreted these findings as suggestive that BPD patients may improve in later middle-age. Others take a less sanguine view, however, and express concern that diagnostic criteria may simply be insensitive to BPD in late life.

Rosowsky and Gurian (1991), for example, examined the records of eight elderly patients identified as BPD by clinicians experienced with geriatric populations who had had extensive contact with the patients. In this study, the patients were genuinely older adults, ranging in age from 64 to 85. The researchers applied both the DIB-R and the DSM-III-R criteria to the identified individuals. Not a single one was identified as having BPD by the DIB-R and only two were identified by the DSM-III-R. They concluded that the DIB-R and the DSM criteria were invalid with this specific aged population. Careful analysis of their data revealed that certain domains of the DIB-R and certain DSM criteria *were* sensitive to the sample. In particular, they found that difficulties with interpersonal relationships and social adaptation, affective dysregulation and anger were clearly impaired relative to age-matched, but non-BPD controls. In contrast, they found that neither the domains of impulsivity nor the criteria regarding identity disturbance were sensitive enough to discriminate BPD patients in late life.

Agronin and Maletta (2000) addressed the general lack of research on personality disorders in late life, and pointed to a number of reasons that such research is difficult to conduct, including the relatively recent development of diagnostic criteria and the necessity of reviewing the entire life history of the patient. They also pointed to a number of specific difficulties in assessing BPD in late life. First, a pattern of unstable and intense interpersonal relationships may be hard to assess in late life, when the attenuation of social relationships and losses due to death may make it difficult to ascertain the degree to which it has been a chronic and pervasive problem. Second, they pointed out that identity disturbance is less relevant in late life, and that it is unclear exactly how it would present, since defining life choices regarding sexual orientation, marriage/family and career are no longer relevant. Finally, they note, as above, that levels of impulsivity appear to decline in late life. However, they point out that the mode of expression of self-harming behaviors may be quite different in late life, and that the examples provided in the DSM-IV may not be applicable to geriatric populations. They suggest that better examples might include things like non-compliance with medical treatments, polypharmacy, and disordered eating.

ETIOLOGY

Genetic Vulnerability and Neurobiological Findings. There is considerable evidence that BPD is heritable. One twin study of personality disorders (Torgersen, Lygren, Oien et al., 2000) found concordance rates of 7% in dizygotic twins, but 35% in monozygotic twins, suggesting a substantial genetic component. They calculated the heritability of BPD at 69%. Skodol, Siever, Livesley et al. (2002) suggested that BPD may be the result of several different clusters of heritable traits, the most important of which is probably emotional dysregulation. They noted that the central psychobiological domains of BPD include impulsive aggression, which is associated with reduced serotonergic activity, and affective instability, which is associated with increased responsiveness of the cholinergic systems.

Both structural and functional neuroimaging studies have also suggested a clear biological etiology to BPD. A number of studies have
pointed to dysregulation of the frontal and limbic brain regions, which
together are responsible broadly for both impulse control and affective
regulation. For example, Schmahl and colleagues (Schmahl, Elzinga,
Vermetten et al., 2003; Schmahl, Vermetten, Elzinga et al., 2004) have
found evidence that the anterior cingulate cortex fails to activate fully in
women with BPD when they are exposed to stressful memories of abandonment or childhood abuse. Other studies have found evidence of
structural and metabolic changes in the limbic system, such as reduced
volume of the hippocampus and amygdala (Driessen, Herrmann, Stahl
et al., 2000) along with increased metabolic activity in the amygdala under emotional arousal conditions (Donegan, Sanislow, Blumberg et al.,
2003). There is also evidence of stress hormone (cortisol) induced
changes in the brain systems of women with BPD that are very similar
to those seen in chronic PTSD (Rinne, de Kloet, Wouters et al., 2002)
and strongly suggest chronic hyperresponsiveness of the hypothalamic-pituitary-adrenal (HPA) axis.

Of course, while genetic studies certainly point unequivocally to etiology, the other biological findings cited above could simply be descriptive of the symptoms experienced by patients with BPD in the here
and now. That is, such biological changes may be concomitant with the
affective instability BPD patients experience, rather than causal. Knowing that there are considerable biological and neurological correlates of
the borderline syndrome is helpful, however, when it comes to
maintaining empathy and planning treatment.

Childhood Experience and Trauma

Of much more clear-cut etiological relevance to BPD is childhood
experience and, in particular, childhood trauma, abuse and neglect.
Zanarini and colleagues (Zanarini, Williams, Lewis et al., 1997;
Zanarini, Yong, Frankenburg et al., 2002) found that of 358 patients
with BPD, 91% reported having been abused and 92% reported having
been neglected before the age of 18. Moreover, BPD patients (relative
to other personality disorders) were significantly more likely to have
been emotionally and physically abused by a caretaker and sexually
abused by a non-caretaker. They were also significantly more likely to
have had a caretaker withdraw from them emotionally, or treat them
inconsistently. Finally, the severity of reported childhood sexual
abuse was correlated with the severity of borderline pathology and

psychosocial impairment in adulthood. McLean and Gallop (2003) found that both BPD and complex PTSD were far more likely in women reporting early-onset sexual abuse than late-onset sexual abuse. Goodman and Yehuda (2002) traced how childhood trauma could impact brain morphology, serotonergic responsivity and HPA axis reactivity in ways that are consistent with the various symptom clusters of BPD, including impulsive aggression, dissociation, identity disturbance and affective instability. In a recent review, Bradley, Jenei and Westen (2005) note that a substantial body of research has confirmed that there is a link between BPD and childhood abuse and neglect. They also found that while childhood sexual abuse contributed to the prediction of BPD symptoms over and above family environment, other family factors such as instability partially mediated that effect.

One potential mediating mechanism between childhood abuse/neglect and adult BPD is that early experience alters one's worldview and basic beliefs about the self. Butler, Brown, Beck and Grisham (2002) found evidence that BPD patients hold numerous dysfunctional beliefs reflecting themes of dependency, helplessness, distrust, fears of rejection/abandonment and fear of losing emotional control. Giesen-Bloo and Arntz (2005) also found that BPD patients hold inflexible and maladaptive beliefs. They tend to view the world as malevolent, and themselves as unworthy and incapable.

Graybar and Boutilier (2002) sounded a cautionary note, however, and pointed out that childhood abuse is neither necessary nor sufficient to cause BPD. Many victims of childhood abuse do not grow up to suffer from BPD, and a substantial minority of BPD patients report no significant childhood abuse. They point to other, non-traumatic pathways, including temperamental vulnerability and neurological deficits.

In summary, it seems that the best way to conceptualize the etiology of BPD is that a powerful diathesis (a temperament highly prone to affective lability, sometimes clearly verging on bipolar spectrum disorders) combines with stressors such as childhood trauma (which can also result in chronic, complex PTSD). The trauma is neither necessary nor sufficient, but does have implications for severity in a dose-response relationship—the more severe and long-lasting the trauma, the more severe the BPD pathology is likely to be. Together, these two major etiological factors result in changes at a number of levels, including the biological, cognitive, experiential and behavioral. In the end, BPD patients are left with wildly dysregulated emotions, distorted cognitions, severe social skills deficits, and few coping strategies they can count on.

EFFECTIVE TREATMENTS

Affective Instability

The Role of Medication. Several classes of psychotropic medication have proven to be quite useful in managing some of the more distressing symptoms of BPD (see Mohan, 2002 for a review). Mood stabilizers/anticonvulsants have proved to reduce affective lability as well as behavioral impulsivity. Randomized controlled trials have supported the use of lithium (Links, 1990), carbamazapine/tegretol (Cowdry & Gardner, 1988), divalproex sodium/depakote (Hollander, Allen, Lopez et al., 2001) and lamotrigine/lamictal (Pinto & Akiskal, 1998). Antidepressants, especially the SSRIs and the MAOIs, are also useful, especially in reducing symptoms related to anger/irritability, and not just in cases where there are significant depressive symptoms (e.g., Coccaro & Kavoussi, 1997; Cowdry & Gardner, 1988). In severe cases, there is good reason to consider the use of antipsychotic medications, especially some of the newer generation medications (e.g., Olanzapine/Zyprexa) that have more tolerable side-effect profiles and secondary mood stabilizing attributes (e.g., Schulz, Camlin, Berry & Jesberger, 1999).

The main difficulty with pharmacotherapy for patients with BPD is that they may be highly resistant to taking psychiatric medication. They may be loathe to "depend" on a substance, and may reject any positive effects as "false" because they feel so discordant with their normal state. Careful explanation of the mechanism of action of various medications can help, as can pointing out that there is no "black market" for Zoloft or Tegretol because they are not "mood enhancing" drugs. That is, they only work when there is an underlying problem that needs to be fixed.

Distress Tolerance and Affect Regulatory Skills. While pharmacotherapy can go a long way toward relieving some of the more acute affective distress and impulsivity, psychotherapeutic interventions are still necessary. BPD patients often have very little tolerance for distress (Linehan, 1993) and few normative skills for regulating affective experience. Unfortunately, the strategies they turn to (e.g., dissociation, self-mutilation, binge eating, or substance use) are powerful anodynes in the short term. Going for a walk, taking a bath, or drawing a picture simply doesn't give the same immediate and powerful relief. Therefore, it is crucial to help BPD patients understand the tradeoff between short-term relief and long-term exacerbation of the very symptoms they are trying to escape. Most BPD patients quickly grasp the long-term costs of such behaviors. They know that they end up feeling worse. They simply can't think of alternatives in the moment.

Relationship Instability

Using the Therapeutic Relationship. The core component of a corrective therapeutic experience for patients with BPD is probably *validation* (Linehan, 1993). This one strategy allows the caregiver to maintain empathy and helps the BPD patient develop a trusting, constructive relationship with the caregiver. It is certainly true that the behavior of people with BPD is often highly maladaptive, and often brings about exactly the social rejection and abandonment by caretakers that they most fear. However, it is also the case that they are genuinely in enormous pain, and are truly doing the best they can with the skill set they have to cope with life and manage their emotions and their social relationships. *Validating* their pain–that is, acknowledging the legitimacy of their feelings and empathizing with their distress, confusion, frustration and even rage, often goes a long way towards calming them down. One does not have to *agree* that their emotional response is proportional or even appropriate to the events in question, but it is crucial to acknowledge their experience and to try to understand how they interpreted the events. This is the first necessary step in helping them to recognize and change their distorted beliefs and maladaptive behaviors. Caretakers must remember that patients with BPD often came from genuinely neglectful or abusive origins, and that this has sensitized them to the least hint of maltreatment.

One useful strategy is to warn BPD patients up front that caregivers are human, and will, therefore, make mistakes. It is important that the patient agrees to let the caregiver know when they feel angry or wounded, so that the caregiver can apologize for any missteps and the patient and caregiver can work together to try to avoid similar incidents from reoccurring.

Addressing Social Skills Deficits. When BPD patients "act-up" it is often because they have misinterpreted some aspect of the social environment in a way that is consistent with a core maladaptive belief (Newman, 1998). Caregivers should try to explore and understand the perspective of the patient–that is, how they perceived and interpreted a series of events–in order to make sense of the patient's maladaptive behavior. Caregivers should also actively model adaptive social problem-solving.

Self-Harming and Suicidality

One of the most disturbing and frightening aspects of borderline personality disorder for most clinicians is the management of self-injurious behavior, including non-suicidal self-injury (e.g., self-mutilation such as "cutting" and burning) and suicide attempts. While there is evidence that these behaviors decline substantially in later life (e.g., Stevenson, Meares & Comerford, 2003), there is also reason to think that they may simply be expressed in other, more subtle ways (e.g., Agronin & Maletta, 2000). These behaviors are easily interpreted by care providers and family as "manipulative acting out" and are a primary reason many therapists are reluctant to work with patients with BPD. Indeed, para-suicidal behavior is the single best predictor of death by suicide (Gunnell & Frankel, 1994).

Brown, Comtois and Linehan (2002) examined the self-reported reasons for non-suicidal self-injury in a sample of 75 women with BPD. They found that BPD patients engage in self-injury primarily to *manage out-of-control affect*. That is, self-harming behavior provided a powerful distraction from painful emotions, but also allowed the individual to *express* emotions, especially anger, in a powerful, but private way and could be used to normalize emotional experience. It was also reported to be a way to punish the self for perceived failings. Stanley and Brodsky (2005) conceptualize self-injurious behavior primarily as a means to *self-regulation*. Paris (2005) also found that self-mutilation is most likely to be a means of regulating dysphoric affect and coping with dissociative states, although it can also be used as a way to communicate distress.

Ironically, self-mutilatory behavior is often assumed to be manipulative–a way of punishing or expressing anger towards those the BPD patient perceives as having injured them, but this is quite inconsistent with the actual clinical phenomenon. Most self-injurious behavior is carried out in secret, inflicted on hidden parts of the body, and rarely disclosed to a caregiver unless the patient is directly confronted. BPD patients assume, quite rightly, that if they reveal self-injurious behavior, it will quickly become a target of treatment, and most are reluctant to give up this highly efficacious (though clearly maladaptive and counter-therapeutic) strategy for regulating their own distress.

PSYCHOTHERAPY OUTCOME STUDIES

Very few randomized controlled trials have assessed the efficacy of therapeutic interventions for BPD. Dialectical behavior therapy (DBT), a variant of cognitive behavioral therapy, has the most empirical support, with seven well-controlled trials (see Lieb, Zanarini, Schmahl et al., 2004). DBT is a highly comprehensive treatment program that includes both individual and group therapy, skills training, and weekly meetings of therapeutic staff for support and consultation (Lieb et al., 2004; Linehan, 1993). An open trial of cognitive therapy (CT) in which patients received weekly individual therapy (and therapists participated in monthly group consultation and support) also showed promising results including significant and clinically important decreases on measures of suicide ideation, hopelessness, depression, number of borderline symptoms and dysfunctional beliefs at termination and 18-month assessment interviews (Brown, Newman, Charlesworth et al., 2004; Layden, Newman, Freeman & Morse, 1993). Finally, a very recent RCT comparing schema focused cognitive therapy to psychodynamic therapy found the CT intervention to be significantly more effective (Arntz, 2005).

BPD IN NURSING HOMES AND GERIATRIC SERVICES

While comprehensive treatment programs for BPD are probably the ideal, they may be quite unrealistic for late-life patients who are residents of nursing homes or are otherwise receiving geriatric care. Rosowksy and Gurian (1992) point out that the symptoms of BPD in elderly patients have a considerable impact on systems of care for geriatric patients. For example, they note that food refusal, non-compliance and the active sabotage of medical care may be geriatric variants of self-harming behaviors. Moreover, disturbed interpersonal relationships can wreak havoc in a nursing home setting. They note that elderly patients with BPD may still show the typical vacillation between overvaluing and demeaning care providers, including nursing staff, occupational therapists and social workers. Affective instability and mismanaged anger in the patient can result in insulting behavior, excessive litigiousness and conflicts with authority. This can lead to considerable resentment and frustration on the part of caregivers, who may feel trapped by basic ethical and legal constraints into complying with outrageous requests and excessive demands made by such patients. Moreover, BPD patients can often cause "splits" or conflict between caregivers, who may find themselves either defending or vilifying the patient. It is important in such cases to view the conflict as stemming from the BPD pathology, and to ensure frequent case consultation among caregivers to minimize such friction.

Trappler and Backfield (2001) tracked the impact of three different BPD patients who were older than 50 on an inpatient psychiatric unit. They note that the actual losses associated with aging (of significant others or of physical health) are likely to trigger decompensation in elderly patients with BPD. They raise the concern that frailty, loss, and fear of abandonment may be inadvertently reinforced in institutional care settings, resulting in heightened somatization and protracted hospital stays. Fear of loss and fear of abandonment are developmentally normative for many geriatric patients–but such normative concerns are grossly exaggerated in the BPD patient, and may lead to frantic, demanding and antagonistic behavior with caregivers, which is easily misinterpreted as manipulative, hostile or cruel. Caregivers must be free to set appropriate limits, but should also recognize the genuine terror that an elderly BPD patient may be experiencing.

Himelick and Walsh (2002) also reviewed how BPD pathology manifests itself in long-term care settings, and pointed to the serious problems BPD patients often experience in relating to nursing and therapeutic staff. They make excellent recommendations for how social workers can develop intervention strategies and serve as intermediaries between the BPD patient and the staff, helping to minimize the common polarization or "splitting" that often occurs in such cases. They emphasize the need for validating the BPD patients' physical and emotional pain and needs, while simultaneously encouraging caregiving staff to set appropriate limits and boundaries with such patients. They also recommend that specific behavioral contingencies be established that will encourage appropriate self-care, and will discourage the patient from sabotaging medical interventions. For example, a patient might be reinforced for eating, or leaving an IV in place, with extra time with a favorite staff member. Attention and support then become contingent on appropriate, adaptive behavior, rather than the patient receiving extra care in response to maladaptive behavior. Educating the caregiving staff about the goals and utility of such plans is crucial, lest they view the plan as "rewarding" or "caving in to" a problematic patient.

In the end, the interventions with geriatric BPD patients have a similar goal as the interventions with younger patients. Caregivers must validate the very real losses, traumas and emotional pain the patient is experiencing, as well as their (often well-founded) fear of abandonment. They must then find ways to help the patient understand that more adaptive, consistent behavior will actually result in less distress in the long run as caregivers are better able to meet their needs. The losses of old age are legion in the best of circumstances. When they are magnified by the BPD patients' *history* of loss, trauma and neglect, by their vulnerability to affective disorder, and by a genuine lack of adaptive coping skills, it is no surprise that such patients would engage in desperate measures to manage their pain and get their needs met. It is crucial that caregivers maintain their empathy for these fragile patients, while still demanding and setting the stage for adaptive change.

REFERENCES

Agronin, M.E. & Maletta, G. (2000). Personality disorders in late life: Understanding and overcoming the gap in research. *American Journal of Geriatric Psychiatry, 8(1)*, 4-18.

Akiskal, H.S. (1981). Subaffective disorders: Dysthymic, cyclothymic and bipolar II disorders in the "borderline" realm. *Psychiatric Clinics of North America, 4*, 25-46.

Akiskal, H.S. (1985). Borderline: An adjective in search of a noun. *Journal of Clinical Psychiatry, 46*, 41-48.

Akiskal, H.S., Hirschfield, R.M.A. & Yerevanian, B.I. (1983). The relationship of personality to affective disorders. *Archives of General Psychiatry, 40*, 801-810.

Akiskal, H.S., Walker, P., Puzantian, V., King, D., Rosenthal, T.L. & Dranon, M. (1983). Bipolar outcome in the course of depressive illness. Phenomenologic, familial and pharmacologic predictors. *Journal of Affective Disorders, 5*, 115-128.

American Psychiatric Association (1994) DSM-IV: Diagnostic and statistical manual for mental disorders, 4th Edition. American Psychiatric Association, Washington, DC.

Arntz, A. (2005, September). Schema-focused therapy and psychodynamic therapy: A comparison. Paper presented at the German Behavior Therapy Association conference; Status and Perspectives of Behaviour Therapy: An International Point of View, Frankfurt, Germany.

Bradley, R., Jenei, J. & Westen, D. (2005). Etiology of borderline personality disorder: Disentangling the contributions of intercorrelated antecedents. *The Journal of Nervous and Mental Disease, 193(1)*, 24-31.

Brown, G.K., Newman, C.F., Charlesworth, S.E., Crits-Christoph, P. & Beck, A.T. (2004). An open clinical trial of cognitive therapy for borderline personality disorder. *Journal of Personality Disorders, 18(3)*, 257-271.

Brown, M.Z., Comtois, K.A. & Linehan, M.M. (2002). Reasons for suicide attempts and nonsuicidal self-injury in women with borderline personality disorder. *Journal of Abnormal Psychology, 111(1)*, 198-202.

Butler, A.C., Brown, G.K., Beck, A.T. & Grisham, J.R. (2002). Assessment of dysfunctional beliefs in borderline personality disorder. *Behaviour Research and Therapy, 40*, 1231-1240.

Coccaro, E.F. & Kavoussi, R.J. (1997). Fluoxetine and impulsive aggressive behavior in personality disordered subjects. *Archives of General Psychiatry, 54(12)*, 1081-1088.

Cowdry, R.W. & Gardner, D.L. (1988). Pharmacotherapy of borderline personality disorder. Alprazolam, carbamazepine, trifluoperazine, and tranylcypromine. *Archives of General Psychiatry, 45(2),* 111-119.

Donegan, N.H., Sanislow, C.A., Blumberg, H.P., Fulbright, R.K., Lacadie, C., Skudlarsky, P., Gore, J.C., Olson, I.R., McGlashan, T.H., & Wexler, B.E. (2003). Amygdala hyperreactivity in borderline personality disorder: Implications for emotional dysregulation. *Biological Psychiatry, 54(11),* 1284-1293.

Driessen, M., Herrmann, J., Stahl, K., Zwaan, M., Meier, S., Hill, A., Osterheider, M. & Petersen, D. (2000). Magnetic resonance imaging volumes of the hippocampus and the amygdale in women with borderline personality disorder and early traumatization. *Archives of General Psychiatry, 57(12),* 1115-1122.

Giesen-Bloo, J. & Arntz, A. (2005). World assumptions and the role of trauma in borderline personality disorder. *Journal of Behavior Therapy and Experimental Psychiatry. Special Issue: Cognition and Emotion in Borderline Personality Disorder, 36(3),* 197-208.

Goodman, M. & Yehuda, R. (2002). The relationship between psychological trauma and borderline personality disorder. *Psychiatric Annals, 32(6),* 337-345.

Graybar, S.R. & Boutilier, L.R. (2002). Nontraumatic pathways to borderline personality disorder. *Psychotherapy: Theory, Research, Practice, Training, 39(2),* 152-162.

Gunderson, J.G. & Sabo, A.N. (1993a). The phenomenological and conceptual interface between borderline personality disorder and PTSD. *American Journal of Psychiatry, 150(1),* 19-27.

Gunderson, J.G. & Sabo, A.N. (1993b). Borderline personality disorder and PTSD: Reply. *American Journal of Psychiatry, 150(12),* 1906-1907.

Gunnell, D. & Frankel, S. (1994). Prevention of suicide: Aspirations and evidence. *British Medical Journal, 308,* 1227-1233.

Himelick, A.J. & Walsh, J. (2002). Nursing home residents with borderline personality traits: Clinical social work interventions. *Journal of Gerontological Social Work, 37(1),* 49-63.

Hollander, E., Allen, A., Lopez, R.P., Bienstock, C.A., Grossman, R., Siever, L.J., Merkatz, L. & Stein, D.J. (2001). A preliminary double-blind, placebo-controlled trial of divalproex sodium in borderline personality disorder. *Journal of Clinical Psychiatry, 62(3),* 199-203.

Kudler, H.S. (1993). Borderline personality disorder and PTSD. *American Journal of Psychiatry, 150(12),* 1906.

Layden, M.A., Newman, C.F., Freeman, A. & Morse, S.B. (1993). *Cognitive Therapy of Borderline Personality Disorder,* Psychology practitioner guidebooks. Needham Heights, MA, US: Allyn & Bacon.

Lieb, K., Zanarini, M.C., Schmahl, C., Linehan, M.M. & Bohus, M. (2004). Borderline personality disorder. *Lancet, 364,* 453-461.

Linehan, M.M. (1993). *Cognitive-behavioral treatment of borderline personality disorder.* NY, London: The Guilford Press.

Links, P. (1990). Lithium therapy for borderline patients. *Journal of Personality Disorders, 4,* 173-181.

McGill, C.A. (2004). The boundary between borderline personality disorder and bipolar disorder: Current concepts and challenges. *Canadian Journal of Psychiatry, 49(8),* 551-556.

McLean, L.M. & Gallop, R. (2003). Implications of childhood sexual abuse for adult borderline personality disorder and complex posttraumatic stress disorder. *American Journal of Psychiatry, 160(2),* 369-371.

Mohan, R. (2002). Treatments for borderline personality disorder: Integrating evidence into practice. *International Review of Psychiatry, 14,* 42-51.

Newman, C.F. (1998). Cognitive therapy for borderline personality disorder. In Vandecreek, L., Knapp, S. & Jackson, T. (Eds.) *Innovations in Clinical Practice: A Source Book, Vol. 16* (pp. 17-38). Sarasota, FL, US: Professional Resource Press/Professional Resource Exchange, Inc.

Paris, J. (2002). Chronic suicidality among patients with borderline personality disorder. *Psychiatric Services, 53(6),* 738-742.

Paris, J. & Zweig-Frank, H. (2001). A 27-year follow-up of patients with borderline personality disorder. *Comprehensive Psychiatry, 42(6),* 482-487.

Perugi, G., Akiskal, H.S., Lattanzi, L., Cecconi, D., Mastrocinque, C., Patronelli, A. et al. (1998). The high prevalence of soft bipolar II features in atypical depression. *Comprehensive Psychiatry, 39,* 63-71.

Perugi, G., Toni, C., Travierso, M.C. & Akiskal, H.S. (2003). The role of cyclothymia in atypical depression: Toward a data-based reconceptualization of the borderline-bipolar II connection. *Journal of Affective Disorders, 73,* 87-98.

Pinto, O.C. & Akiskal, H.S. (1998). Lamotrigine as a promising approach to borderline personality: An open case series without concurrent DSM-IV major mood disorder. *Journal of Affective Disorders, 51(3),* 333-343.

Reich, J., Nduaguba, M. & Yates, W. (1988). Age and sex distribution of DSM-III personality cluster traits in a community population. *Comprehensive Psychiatry, 29(3),* 298-303.

Rinne, T., de Kloet, E.R., Wouters, L., Goekoop, J.G., DeRijk, R.H. & van den Brink, W. (2002). Hyperresponsiveness of hypothalamic-pituitary-adrenal axis to combined dexamethasone/corticotrophin-releasing hormone challenge in female borderline personality disorder subjects with a history of sustained childhood abuse. *Biological Psychiatry, 52,* 1102-1112.

Rosowsky, E. & Gurian, B. (1991). Borderline personality disorder in late life. *International Psychogeriatrics, 3(1),* 39-52.

Rosowsky, E. & Gurian, B. (1992). Impact of borderline personality disorder in late life on systems of care. *Hospital and Community Psychiatry, 43(4),* 386-389.

Schmahl, C.G., Elzinga, B.M., Vermetten, E., Sanislow, C., McGlashan, T.H. & Bremner, J.D. (2003). Neural correlates of memories of abandonment in women with and without borderline personality disorder. *Biological Psychiatry, 54,* 142-151.

Schmahl, C.G., Vermetten, E., Elzinga, B.M. & Bremner, J.D. (2004). A positron emission tomography study of memories of childhood abuse in borderline personality disorder. *Biological Psychiatry, 55,* 759-765.

Schulz, S.C., Camlin, K.L., Berry, S.A. & Jesberger, J.A. (1999). Olanzapine safety and efficacy in patients with borderline personality disorder and comorbid dysthymia. *Biological Psychiatry, 46(10),* 1429-1435.

Shea, M.T., Zlotnick, C. & Weisberg, R.B. (1999). Commonality and specificity of personality disorder profiles in subjects with trauma histories. *Journal of Personality Disorders, 13,* 199-210.

Skodol, A.E., Siever, L.J., Livesley, W.J., Gunderson, J.G., Pfohl, B. & Widiger, T.A. (2002). The borderline diagnosis II: Biology, genetics, and clinical course. *Biological Psychiatry, 51(12),* 951-963.

Smith, D.J., Muir, W.J., & Blackwood, D.H.R. (2005). Borderline personality disorder characteristics in young adults with recurrent mood disorders: A comparison of bipolar and unipolar depression. *Journal of Affective Disorders, 87,* 17-23.

Smith, D.J., Muir, W.J., & Blackwood, D.H.R. (2004). Is borderline personality disorder part of the bipolar spectrum? *Harvard Review of Psychiatry, 12(3),* 133-139.

Stanley, B. & Brodsky, B.S. (2005). Suicidal and self-injurious behavior in borderline personality disorder: A self-regulation model. In Gunderson, J. & Hoffman, P. (Eds.) *Understanding and Treating Borderline Personality Disorder: A Guide for Professionals and Families* (pp. 43-63). Washington, DC: American Psychiatric Publishing, Inc.

Stevenson, J., Meares, R. & Comerford, A. (2003). Diminished impulsivity in older patients with borderline personality disorder. *American Journal of Psychiatry, 160(1),* 165-166.

Swartz, M., Blazer, D., George, L. & Winfield, I. (1990). Estimating the prevalence of borderline personality disorder in the community. *Journal of Personality Disorders, 4(3),* 257-272.

Torgersen, S., Lygren, S., Oien, P.A., Skre, I., Onstad, S., Edvardsen, J., Tambs, K. & Kringlen, E. (2000). A twin study of personality disorders. *Comprehensive Psychiatry, 41(6),* 416-425.

Trappler, B. & Backfield, J. (2001). Clinical characteristics of older psychiatric inpatients with borderline personality disorder. *Psychiatric Quarterly, 72(1),* 29-40.

Widiger, T.A. & Weissman, M.M. (1991). Epidemiology of borderline personality disorder. *Hospital and Community Psychiatry, 42(10),* 1015-1021.

Zanarini, M.C., Frankenburg, F.R., Dubo, E.D., Sickel, A.E., Trikha, A., Levin, A. & Reynolds, R. (1998). Axis I comorbidity of borderline personality disorder. *American Journal of Psychiatry, 115,* 1733-1739.

Zanarini, M.C., Gunderson, J.G., Frankenburg, F.R. & Chauncey, D.L. (1989). The Revised Diagnostic Interview for Borderlines: discriminating BPD from other axis II disorders. *Journal of Personality Disorders, 3,* 10-18.

Zanarini, M.C., Williams, A.A., Lewis, R.E., Reich, R.B., Vera, S.C., Marino, M.F., Levin, A., Yong, L. & Frankenburg, F. (1997). Reported pathological childhood experiences associated with the development of borderline personality disorder. *American Journal of Psychiatry, 154,* 1101-1106.

Zanarini, M.C., Yong, L., Frankenburg, F.R., Hennen, J., Reich, D., Marino, M.F. & Vujanovic, A. (2002). Severity of reported childhood sexual abuse and its relationship to severity of borderline psychopathology and psychosocial impairment among borderline patients. *Journal of Nervous and Mental Disorders, 190,* 381-387.

Zlotnick, C., Johnson, D.M., Yen, S., Battle, C.L., Sanislow, C.A., Skodol, A.E., Grilo, C.M., McGlashan, T.H., Gunderson, J.G., Bender, D.S., Zanarini, M.C. & Shea, M.T. (2003). Clinical features and impairment in women with Borderline Personality Disorder (BPD) with Posttraumatic Stress Disorder (PTSD), BPD without PTSD, and other personality disorders with PTSD. *The Journal of Nervous and Mental Disease, 191(11),* 706-713.

doi:10.1300/J074v19n01_11

Conclusions

Victor J. Malatesta, PhD

This special volume attempted to offer a comprehensive overview for the health professional who is seeking a greater depth of understanding with respect to the study of mental problems in general, and how these issues pertain specifically to women and the aging process. A second goal of this project was to offer the practicing therapist and counselor a research update and a broad clinical perspective offered by seasoned clinicians. Utilizing current psychiatric nosology as a framework, we attempted to focus on the mental health problems of older women by emphasizing description and diagnosis, prevalence, etiology, assessment and treatment, and suggestions for future research. We hope that our efforts have moved the ball a little further down the field.

There are many questions that remain with respect to women, aging and their mental health problems. Questions remain about the trajectory of many mental health problems in older women. Under-diagnosis and the challenge of differential diagnosis are common concerns across domains. While there is clarity about the unique challenges faced by older women with cognitive complaints, we are only gearing up to address the greater number and impact of older women who display alcohol use disorders. Although much is known about older women who suffer from schizophrenia, questions remain about how best to provide for these women who are at risk for neglect and who are overrepresented in boarding homes and among the homeless. While 50% of older adults experience their first episode of major depression in the latter part of

[Haworth co-indexing entry note]: "Conclusions." Malatesta, Victor J. Co-published simultaneously in *Journal of Women & Aging* (The Haworth Press, Inc.) Vol. 19, No. 1/2, 2007, pp. 193-196; and: *Mental Health Issues of Older Women: A Comprehensive Review for Health Care Professionals* (ed: Victor J. Malatesta) The Haworth Press, Inc., 2007, pp. 193-196. Single or multiple copies of this article are available for a fee from The Haworth Document Delivery Service [1-800-HAWORTH, 9:00 a.m. - 5:00 p.m. (EST). E-mail address: docdelivery@haworthpress.com].

doi:10.1300/J074v19n01_12

life, there are questions about how best to disentangle the range of medical and psychosocial factors that will affect the course and severity of the disorder.

With respect to anxiety disorders, there are questions that pertain to helping older women negotiate the various biological and psychosocial stressors that give rise to anxiety symptoms and their disorders. Much work remains to be done within the area of posttraumatic stress disorder (PTSD) and older women. Under-diagnosis is common, and there is a question about how to support older women who are unaccustomed to and uncomfortable with revealing their histories of trauma. Relatedly, the issue of dissociative disorders in older women is an important topic that is worthy of additional study, and again raises questions about under-diagnosis, differential diagnosis, and the best treatment avenues. The conceptualization and treatment of sexual problems among older women are in a state of transition. Similarly, an emerging clinical literature indicates the need to study the development and treatment of eating disorders in older women. Many questions remain about the treatment of borderline personality disorder in older women, and how best to address their needs in other life-care settings, including nursing homes. Finally, we are only beginning to observe the development of individually tailored mental health treatments for older adult women.

A NEED FOR GREATER ATTENTION TO MULTIETHNIC, MULTICULTURAL AND SEXUAL MINORITY ISSUES

This project has also revealed general areas in need of greater clinical and research attention. Most notable is the need for work that addresses the mental health issues of older women of color, of various socioeconomic levels, and of ethnic groups that are growing rapidly (e.g., Latino, Asian). While available research suggests that the prevalence of mental health problems for these older women is similar (if not greater, for example, with respect to older women in poverty), their coping patterns and use of services are likely to be different (e.g., Howell & McEvatt, 2005). Recent work has addressed some of these multiethnic, multicultural and socioeconomic issues (e.g., Howell & McEvatt, 2005; Mjelde-Mossey & Walz, 2006; Slater et al., 2003; West et al., 2004). Relatedly, there is need for attention to the mental health issues of lesbian and bisexual older women (see Hughes, Smith, & Dan, 2003; Mathy & Kerr, 2004). Taken together, periodicals like the *Journal of Women & Aging* offer a special forum for this work.

A NEED FOR MORE TRAINING AND CONTINUING EDUCATION IN WORKING WITH OLDER WOMEN

An ongoing issue is the need for additional training and continuing education in the field of aging. Although practitioners are interested in working with older adults, fewer than 30% of practicing psychologists report having had any graduate course work in geropsychology, and fewer than 20% have had a supervised practicum or internship experience with older adults (Qualls, Segal, Norman, Niederehe, & Gallagher-Thompson, 2002). My impression is that nursing and social work, which have a longer and greater tradition of working with older adults, have done a better job in this area. While psychology has been involved in the field of aging for a number of years (see Malatesta, 1980, 1985), a recent positive development has been the publication by the American Psychological Association of General Guidelines for Psychological Practice in working with older adults (see American Psychological Association, 2004).

In conclusion, the authors and I look forward to continuing and expanding our clinical and research work in this important area. We also look forward to corroborating with and sharing our efforts with our colleagues. Obviously, we all share the same goal of providing older women and men alike the most sensitive and most effective mental health care available.

REFERENCES

American Psychological Association (2004). Guidelines for psychological practice with older adults. *American Psychologist, 59,* 236-260.

Howell, L. C., & McEvatt, L. (2005). Urban black women at midlife: A counseling perspective. *Journal of Women & Aging, 17,* 43-57.

Hughes, T. L., Smith, C., & Dan, A. (Eds.) (2003). *Mental health issues for sexual minority women.* Binghamton, NY: The Haworth Press, Inc.

Malatesta, V. J. (1980). The urban widow: A focus for gerontological study. In J. E. Montgomery & L. H. Walters (Eds.), *Presentations on aging* (pp. 9-21). Athens, GA: University of Georgia Program on Gerontology.

Malatesta, V. J. (1985). Geriatric organic syndromes. In I. D. Turkat (Ed.), *Behavioral case formulation* (pp. 255-307). New York: Plenum.

Mathy, R. M., & Kerr, S. K. (Eds.) (2004). *Lesbian and bisexual women's mental health.* Binghamton, NY: The Haworth Press, Inc.

Mjelde-Mossey, L. A., & Walz, E. (2006). Changing cultural and social environments: Implications for older East Asian women. *Journal of Women & Aging, 18,* 5-20.

Qualls, S. H., Segal, D., Norman, S., Niederehe, G., & Gallagher-Thompson, D. (2002). Psychologists in practice with older adults: Current patterns, sources of training, and need for continuing education. *Professional Psychology: Research and Practice, 33*, 435-442.

Slater, L., Daniel, J. H., & Banks, A. E. (Eds.) (2003). *The complete guide to mental health for women.* Boston: Beacon Press.

West, S. L., Vinokoor, L. C., & Zolnoun, D. (2004). A systematic review of the literature on female sexual dysfunction prevalence and predictors. *Annual Review of Sex Research, 15*, 40-172.

doi:10.1300/J074v19n01_12

About the Contributors

Peter C. Badgio, PhD, received his undergraduate degree from Clark University in 1981 and earned his PhD in Psychology at the University of Pennsylvania in 1986. He served as the Director of Neuropsychology at The Institute of Pennsylvania Hospital until the hospital closed in 1997. He currently maintains a private practice in adult neuropsychology, psychotherapy and psychoanalysis. He teaches psychology interns and psychiatric residents at Pennsylvania Hospital and at the Hospital of the University of Pennsylvania. Dr. Badgio is on the faculty at the Psychoanalytic Center of Philadelphia.

Lynn Brandsma, PhD, is currently Assistant Professor of Psychology at Chestnut Hill College in Philadelphia, PA, where she coordinates the BS/MS program in counseling psychology. She was the founder and Clinical Director of the Lutheran Hospital Eating Disorder Treatment Center in La Crosse, WI. She is a licensed professional counselor and board-certified music therapist, with a clinical specialty in acceptance-based behavioral treatments of obesity and eating disorders.

Faith B. Dickerson, PhD, MPH, is the Director of Psychology at Sheppard Pratt, a not-for-profit psychiatric system in Baltimore, MD, and holds academic appointments in the Departments of Psychiatry at the University of Maryland and Johns Hopkins University. Her research is focused on cognitive and social functioning, psychosocial treatments, and the association between infectious agents and clinical characteristics in persons with serious mental illness.

Elizabeth E. Epstein, PhD, is Associate Professor, Center of Alcohol Studies, and The Graduate School for Applied and Professional Psychology, Rutgers–The State University of New Jersey; and Adjunct Associate Professor, Department of Psychiatry, The University of Medicine and Dentistry of New Jersey. Her research and teaching interests include de-

Available online at http://jwa.haworthpress.com
© 2007 by The Haworth Press, Inc. All rights reserved.
doi:10.1300/J074v19n01_13

velopment and testing of cognitive-behavioral (CBT) models of treatment for alcohol and/or drug-dependent females and males in individual or couples therapy modality, as well as in individual differences and psychiatric comorbidity among substance abusers. She is a grantee of the National Institute on Alcohol Abuse and Alcoholism as well as the National Institute on Drug Abuse. Dr. Epstein also has a part-time private practice focusing primarily on CBT treatment of substance use and mood disorders. With her colleague, Barbara McCrady, she has written *Addictions–A Comprehensive Guidebook* published by Oxford University Press, and is currently writing a CBT treatment manual geared for men, women, and couples.

Kimberly Fischer-Elber, BA, is a doctoral candidate in Clinical Psychology at the Graduate School for Applied and Professional Psychology at Rutgers University. Her research interests include gender differences of alcoholism and alcohol typology. She is currently working on a manuscript on the Type A/B Classification scheme and its applicability to a female sample.

Miriam Franco, MSW, PsyD, is Associate Professor of Sociology at Immaculata University and is a clinical psychologist in private practice. Her research interests focus on women's healthcare and stress and wellness. She has conducted many Stress Reduction and Interactive Imagery workshops for the public and for special health populations. Of particular clinical interest is the application of interactive guided imagery for coping with chronic health conditions.

Reed D. Goldstein, PhD, is currently Clinical Assistant Professor of Psychiatry, University of Pennsylvania School of Medicine and Adjunct, Pennsylvania Hospital Professional Staff in the Department of Psychiatry. Dr. Goldstein is Associate Director, Adult Treatment Inpatient Service, Pennsylvania Hospital, and provides consultations to physicians treating medically and neuropsychiatrically impaired individuals as part of the Consultation-Liaison Service at Pennsylvania Hospital. Previously, he served as Research Associate and Clinical Consultant, Dave Garroway Laboratory for the Study of Depression, Pennsylvania Hospital. Dr. Goldstein has published and made presentations in the areas of depression, personality disorder, neuropsychology, and psychotherapy.

Alan M. Gruenberg, MD, is currently Professor, Department of Psychiatry and Human Behavior, Jefferson Medical College in Philadelphia, PA, and President, Gruenberg & Summers, P.C., a clinical and consulting psychiatric practice in Bryn Mawr, PA, providing diagnostic and longitudinal psychiatric care for children, adolescents, young adults, adults, and seniors. Dr. Gruenberg served on the multiaxial work group for DSM-IV. He was responsible for the text revision for the chapter on multiaxial issues in DSM-IV-TR. He has contributed chapters on Axis III to the recent textbook, *DSM-IV Sourcebook*, Volume 3, and a proposal for multiaxial assessment to the recent volume, *A Research Agenda for DSM-V*. Dr. Gruenberg wrote the chapter on depressive disorders for the Tasman, Kay, Lieberman textbook, *Psychiatry*, first and second editions. He has also published articles on the integration of psychotherapy and pharmacotherapy in treatment of major psychiatric disorders and approaches in pharmacological impasses in treatment.

Melissa Hunt, PhD, earned her BA in Philosophy and Psychology from Yale University in 1987 and her PhD in Clinical Psychology from the University of Pennsylvania in 1996. She currently serves as the Associate Director of Clinical Training in the University of Pennsylvania's Department of Psychology, and as Adjunct Assistant Professor of Community Behavioral Health in the School of Dental Medicine. Her research focuses broadly on the intersection of cognitive change and emotional arousal, and she has published in the areas of depression, stress and coping, phobias and PTSD. In addition to her research, teaching and supervisory responsibilities, she maintains a clinical practice in cognitive-behavioral therapy treating a range of patients with depression, anxiety disorders, trauma and borderline personality disorder.

Richard P. Kluft, MD, practices psychiatry and psychoanalysis in Bala Cynwyd, PA. He is Clinical Professor of Psychiatry, Temple University School of Medicine and on the faculty of the Philadelphia Center for Psychoanalysis, both in Philadelphia, PA. Dr. Kluft has published over 200 scientific articles and book chapters in the dissociative disorders field, and received numerous awards here and abroad for his work in the area. He is currently writing a textbook on the diagnosis and treatment of dissociative disorders.

Stephen Levine, PhD, received his AB degree from the University of California, Berkeley, and his MA and PhD degrees from the University of Illinois, Champaign-Urbana. Currently, Dr. Levine is Clinical Director of The Center for Cognitive & Emotional Well-Being in Wilmington,

DE. He is the past Treasurer and President of the Philadelphia Behavior Association. Dr. Levine worked for over 10 years as a Senior Psychologist in the Psychology Department at the Philadelphia Geriatric Center. He has also been associated for many years with the Anxiety Disorders Clinic at Eastern Psychiatric Institute (now at the University of Pennsylvania). He is married to Roberta Gluck-Levine and has two daughters, Mandara and Kamila.

Zayed Al-Otaiba, MS, is a doctoral candidate in Clinical Psychology at the Psychology Department, Graduate School, New Brunswick at Rutgers–The State University of New Jersey. His research interests are in the areas of addiction treatment and the role of stigma as a barrier to help-seeking. His masters thesis investigates implicit and explicit measures of gender stereotypes of drinking.

Jay Weissman, PhD, obtained his PhD degree in Clinical Psychology from Fairleigh Dickinson University in 1993. Currently, he is in independent practice in Newtown Square, PA, and Wilmington, DE, with a specialty in geriatrics. Formerly, he held the position of Senior Psychologist at the Philadelphia Geriatric Center, where he worked for approximately 20 years. At this time, Dr. Weissman is a consultant at various nursing homes and retirement communities, where he is often a featured speaker, presenting on such topics as anxiety, depression, and dementia in the elderly, as well as running staff development programs. He is a member of several professional organizations, including the Philadelphia Behavior Therapy Association. He resides in Wynnewood, PA, with his wife, Cyd, and their four sons.

Blaise L. Worden, MS, graduated from University of Wisconsin-Madison in 2003. Currently, she works at both the Center of Alcohol Studies and the Anxiety Disorders Clinic at Rutgers University, where she also is a graduate student in the doctoral program for clinical psychology. Her current research focuses on behavioral treatments for alcohol-dependent women, and on mechanisms of change in cognitive-behavioral therapies.

Index